HOLDING SPACE

THE ESSENTIAL GUIDE TO LEADING MEDITATION AND MINDFULNESS PRACTICES

Claire Schneeberger

Audio Samples

Would you like to hear a sample guided meditation?
Access a free audio file or submit your
own audio to share with the community
at the Holding Space website.

holdingspaceguide.com/audio

Book design by Silke Spingies.

ISBN paperback: 979-8-9985573-0-9
ISBN ebook: 979-8-9985573-1-6
LCCN: 2025906630

First edition published in 2025
by Claire Schneeberger, Santa Cruz, CA.

For more information,
email: info@holdingspaceguide.com
www.holdingspaceguide.com

*To all who bring kindness and compassion
to their actions in the world.*

Contents

CHAPTER 1

Why Hold Space? 11

Introduction	13
Holding Space	14
Applications	16
A Focus on Compassion	21
How to Use This Book	24

CHAPTER 2

Fundamentals 27

Fundamental Concepts	28
Benefits of Mindfulness, Meditation, and Compassion Practices	32
Benefits of Group Practice	34

CHAPTER 3

Facilitation Techniques & Tips 39

Fundamentals for Facilitators	40
Facilitation Tips	49

CHAPTER 4

Logistics 55

Meeting Logistics	56
Prepare Yourself	60
Orienting the Group	64
Opening and Closing	66

CHAPTER 5

Practices 81

How to Choose Practices 82

Section 1: Breath-Based Practices 90

1.1. Mindfulness of Breathing 92
1.2. The Zen 10 96
1.3. Finger Tracing 98
1.4. Belly Breathing 100
1.5. Slowing Down the Exhale (aka 4:2:6) 102
1.6. Coherent Breathing 106
1.7. Watching the Cycles of Breathing 110

Section 2: Body-Based Practices 116

2.1. Body Scan 118
2.2. Working with Physical Pain 122
2.3. Walking Meditation 126
2.4. Inside Outside 130
2.5. Cloud Hands 134
2.6. Grounding Like a Tree 136

Section 3: Focused Awareness Practices 140

3.1. Using a Mantra 142
3.2. Gazing 144
3.3. Counting Backward 146

Section 4: Open Awareness Practices 148

4.1. Awareness of Your Environment 150
4.2. Observing Thoughts 152
4.3. Name It to Tame It 156
4.4. Mindful Listening 160

Section 5: Compassion Practices   164

  5.1. Loving-Kindness (Metta)   166
  5.2. Find a Compassionate Image   170
  5.3. Compassion for a Loved One   174
  5.4. Self-Compassion   178
  5.5. Compassionate Touch   184
  5.6. Just Like Me   186
  5.7. Tonglen   190

Closing   194
Acknowledgments   198
Resources   201
Appendix   204
Notes   208
About the Author   213

CHAPTER 1

―――――

Why Hold Space?

"Nothing liberates our greatness like
the desire to help, the desire to serve."

MARIANNE WILLIAMSON

"If you get, give.
If you learn, teach."

MAYA ANGELOU

Introduction

This book is for anyone who wants to lead a group in centering, mindfulness, meditation, compassion, or breathing practices. I'm guessing that you are here because you've experienced the benefits of meditation in some way and felt inspired to share that with others—that was my starting point too. I want you to be able to act on that impulse because the power of shared practice is immense. You can create a space that allows others to tap into their own inner resources and foster a sense of interconnectedness that ripples outward towards greater harmony in the world at large.

It's my premise (and my direct experience) that you don't have to be an expert in meditation or mindfulness to facilitate beneficial group practices. We all possess the ability to hold space for each other. This guidebook will show you how to create space for discovery, healing, growth, insight, connection, and balance. Whether you have five minutes or an hour, you can engage members of your group to create quality connections with themselves and each other.

I want to emphasize that the goal of this book is not to train you to be a meditation teacher or to certify you as a mindfulness expert, though the information here may be a helpful start if you are interested in that path. This book is designed to help a layperson feel confident leading a practice for the benefit of their community. While some experience with meditation or mindfulness is helpful, the essential ingredient is a desire to be of service.

Even though I am a certified teacher of meditation and compassion, when facilitating group practices, I have come to experience myself not as a teacher so much as a *holder of space*—hence the title of this book. As a facilitator I make suggestions and provide guidance, but I know that every participant will have their own unique experience. No experience is better or worse than another. All are equally valid.

A facilitator's role, *your role* if you choose to accept it, is not to impart wisdom but to create the conditions for each participant to access their own truth, wisdom, and strength. This guidebook will show you how.

Holding Space

For me, "holding space" means creating a safe and comfortable environment—a space that allows for relaxation, presence, and the opportunity to simply be. Holding space is a gift to our minds, our bodies, and our nervous systems.

In this frenetic world, however, it is becoming increasingly more difficult to just "be." Life events challenge us. Whether it's a difficult relationship, financial troubles, illness, a medical diagnosis (or lack of a diagnosis), loss, grief, loneliness, discrimination, or injustice—life delivers setbacks.

In addition, news reports continually warn us about the negative impact of our ever-faster lifestyles, including information overload, burnout, anxiety, and existential dread. We also know that technology and the "attention economy" can lead to digital addiction, loneliness, FOMO (fear of missing out), and doomscrolling—all robbing us of opportunities for developing self-knowledge, building meaningful relationships, and doing deep, creative work.

"Almost everything
will work again
if you unplug it
for a few minutes,
including you."

ANNE LAMOTT

Happily, meditation and mindfulness are a proven remedy to all of this. If you care about well-being—about physical, mental, and spiritual health—for yourself and the groups and communities that you are a part of, then you are in the right place. The guidance and specific practices in this book counteract the negative stressors of life and can generate steadiness, strength, creativity, and other positive states.

The focus of this book will not be on the data, facts, and research on mindfulness practice—though you'll find references to excellent information in the Resources section at the end of this book. Knowledge can be great motivation, but actual benefits come from *doing*.

Applications

There are many different settings where groups may want to practice meditation and/or mindfulness. Some may be support groups in a healthcare setting, like the group I lead for women living with cancer. Or you may be part of a community group, a yoga studio, or a workplace interested in fostering well-being. Or you may use these practices to create moments of focus or reflection as part of a class, workshop, or meeting you are leading.

Whether it's your first time, or you have some facilitation experience, you'll find dozens of practices here that apply to a range of situations:

- Leading a mindfulness or meditation group
- Creating focus for a group at the beginning of a meeting
- Settling the energy and creating calm before starting a class
- Setting positive intentions for a workshop or retreat
- Developing connections within a group
- Engaging members in a virtual meeting
- Creating space for relaxation and healing for someone who is stressed
- Providing a moment for reflection at the end of a meeting or class

This guidebook offers you a range of practices you can lead along with advice about how to adapt the practices to your situation. Every group is unique, so I encourage you to experiment and find out what works best in your situation.

MY STORY

My own path of meditation and mindfulness practice has been a winding one.

In my 20s, I was curious about meditation, thinking of it as a pathway to experience expanded consciousness. I attended a class on meditation, and I remember receiving the simple instructions to sit and close my eyes. If you've tried meditation, even once, it will be no surprise to you that nothing special happened. When I closed my eyes, I was aware of a lot of thoughts inside my head—and none of it seemed to represent expanded consciousness. *"Am I doing this right? Why don't I feel anything special? Are other people looking at me? When am I going to feel enlightenment? Sitting on the floor is really uncomfortable..."* I walked away from that class with the assumption that I wasn't good at meditation.

In my 30s, I was running a small business and very stressed out. I knew meditation was supposed to help reduce stress, so I decided to try again. Luckily for me, I found a teacher who helped me understand that meditation is not an instant fix but a lifelong practice of learning to work with the mind—crazy thoughts and all. I started learning different techniques and after dabbling for several years, I established a daily meditation practice.

In my 40s, I gradually increased my meditation time— from five to seven minutes a day, then from eight to 10, to 12. I knew the practice was giving me the clarity and sanity to cope with a career that had me working 60 to

80 hours a week. Based on how much it helped me, I thought about sharing what I was learning with others. But I also knew that meditation was a deep practice, and I was a long way from being an expert. Then I took an eight-week Compassion Cultivation Training™ at Stanford University. During that program I realized that the impossibly high standards I was setting for myself were preventing me from connecting with, and helping, others. I began to teach beginning meditation workshops.

Around that time, I lost two friends to cancer in the span of just a few months. It was difficult, heart-wrenching, filled with love—as they say these days, it was *all the things*. And then someone in my yoga class recommended that I lead the mindful meditation group for a local center that provides services and support to women with cancer—WomenCARE. It was one of those moments that felt like the universe was gifting me the right thing at the right time. This was a way to honor my friends, to help others going through some version of what they had gone through. When I started, I felt my share of imposter syndrome; yet experience taught me that these seemingly simple practices are empowering and transformative. Seeing the positive impact for these women gave me confidence to continue.

In my 50s, I decided to go deeper. I sold my small business and finally had the time to go in new directions. One of those new directions was joining Stanford's Applied Compassion Training,[1] where I spent a year developing my understanding of compassion and applying it to my work. I also completed a meditation teacher training.[2] These programs taught me about the science of compassion and the physiology and neuroscience of both compassion and meditation practices.

The WomenCARE mindful meditation group has given me opportunity to develop and grow. But inevitably, there came a time when I had a conflict with our meeting and needed to find a substitute leader to cover for me. I figured this would be easy because there were many experienced members in the group, but my inquiries were met with reluctance. Even though they had been practicing for years, the idea of leading the group was intimidating. "I'm not an expert," they said. I thought, "if only there was a guidebook to give them confidence and help them feel more prepared, I *know* they could do this." And that's how this book was born.

There have been many moments of doubt along my path, and I hope that what I've learned can be both inspiring and helpful to ease any doubts that you may have. I offer what I have learned and am still learning, not as a set of instructions, but as a suggested starting point for you to try and to ultimately make your own.

A Focus on Compassion

Learning about the principles of compassion and applying them in my life marked a crucial turning point for me. Cultivating compassion within myself, and for myself, gave me the courage to begin sharing mindfulness and meditation practices with others.

I'll go so far as to say that compassion is *the* secret ingredient for success as a facilitator—including compassion for yourself and your entire group. It's the foundation for creating meaningful experiences for your group members. Here are some examples of what compassion as a facilitator looks like.

① Compassionate Acceptance

Holding space for others requires a generosity of spirit and a willingness to accept each person just as they are. Remember, as a facilitator, you don't have to be an expert. Think about it. There's no way you can possibly be an expert on the inner life of another human. You're off the hook! Instead, you are more like a good detective, asking questions and allowing each person's experience to guide them.

In my meditation circle, I like to bring new practices or "experiments" to the group. Afterward I will ask, "How was that for you? Anything to report?" Recently I had someone respond, "I didn't like that at all. It felt bad, and I didn't want to do it, so I did something else instead."

My first instinct was to be defensive—to try to explain why the practice is great and tell them what they missed. But then I remembered, I'm not the expert of their experience—they are! Simply accepting her experience for what it was, I said, "That's so interesting. Everyone has different experiences, and it's useful to learn what works for you and what doesn't. It's great that you found something that worked for you."

Don't tell someone what they *should* be experiencing. Instead, be curious about what they *do* experience. Try to stay in the realm of observation without adding judgments. Learning to accept everyone and everything, with generosity and kindness, is key. It also takes practice, so don't beat yourself up if you slip.

② Embodying Compassion

Facilitating practices offers the benefit of allowing you to practice yourself. Holding space for open exploration, creativity, and connection requires that you shift away from analyzing, judging, comparing, and criticizing and instead cultivate self-compassion, kindness, and acceptance. My Stanford Applied Compassion Training referred to this as a "forever practice," so don't expect it to be easy. It takes self-awareness, but when you make the effort to be present and compassionate you will draw these qualities out in others.

Before you begin, check in with your own intentions.

- Are you ready to let go of your agenda for a particular outcome?
- Are you willing to be human and imperfect?
- Are you committed to noticing and setting aside judgments?

"If we practice mindfulness with judgment, we are growing judgment. If we practice with frustration, we are growing frustration. ... Mindfulness isn't just about paying attention. It's about how we pay attention. True mindfulness involves an attitude of kindness and curiosity."

SHAUNA SHAPIRO,
GOOD MORNING, I LOVE YOU

How to Use This Book

If you picked up this book, I'm guessing that you are already interested in leading group practices, and I hope that this chapter has given you the confidence to carry forward. Depending on your current level of experience, you may want to skip around to the content most relevant to you.

- Chapter 2 contains information on the fundamental concepts and benefits of mindfulness, meditation, and compassion.

- Chapter 3 covers tips for group facilitation.

- Chapter 4 walks you through the logistics of how to prepare and lead practices successfully.

- If you are ready to explore the practices, jump to Chapter 5, where you'll find 27 guided meditations along with an explanation of their benefits.

- Finally, the Resources section at the end of the book provides recommended readings and the Appendix has a sample template for how you might format your group sessions.

———

CHAPTER 2

Fundamentals

This chapter covers some fundamental concepts, including:

- Definitions of mindfulness, meditation, and compassion
- The benefits of practice
- The benefits of group practice

If you are an experienced practitioner, you may want to skim this chapter or jump ahead to Chapter 3 to learn about facilitation.

Fundamental Concepts

When leading practices, it's helpful to be able to clearly explain some key concepts. Here are working definitions of mindfulness, meditation, and compassion that I use. If you want more in-depth information, check out the Resources section at the end of this book for recommended readings.

Mindfulness

Mindfulness is moment-to-moment awareness of one's experience—without judgment. It's not the same as meditation but is a skill that is necessary and used *during* meditation.

The founder of Mindfulness-Based Stress Reduction (MBSR), Jon Kabat-Zinn, defines mindfulness as paying attention in a particular way: 1. on purpose; 2. in the present moment; and 3. nonjudgmentally with openness and curiosity.[3]

Mindfulness is something that can be applied throughout your day. You can be mindful when you eat, when you do the dishes, while you are driving a car, etc. It's a skill that can be developed. Mindfulness is especially crucial during meditation. It allows us to notice the activity of the mind and, with that awareness, begin to direct our mind and change our state of consciousness.

Meditation

Meditation is a practice; it's something that you do—but *not* while you are driving a car! There are many different meditation techniques, which involve drawing awareness within, and learning to focus and quiet the mind. As a result, you may experience peace, calm, creativity, and many other beneficial states.

WHY SO MANY DIFFERENT PRACTICES?

A common misconception about mindfulness and meditation is that it is one thing. Whenever someone says to me, "I'm no good at meditation," I always respond with, "What have you tried?" and "Have you tried other methods?" which often draws the response, "There's more than one way to meditate?!?"

Meditation encompasses many possible methods of practice. It's similar to the concept of sports. If someone told you that they do sports, that's not much information, is it? They could be playing tennis, basketball, or swimming laps in a pool. The same thing is true about meditation. Just as there are many different sports, there are many techniques for meditation.

In a group setting your goal is to provide a range of options, so everyone feels comfortable and able to participate. That's why you'll find 27 practices included in this guidebook. There's no one-size-fits-all way to practice. Given a range of options, everyone can find something they enjoy.

Another thing that meditation and sports share is that different practices build different skills. Some sports build endurance, others build strength or coordination. Similarly, different meditation techniques generate different outcomes—such as focus, relaxation, or connection. Usually, it's some combination of these.

As you gain more experience, you'll learn how to select practices that fit your group and their goals. A good gym teacher wouldn't throw their students into a pool to play water polo if they knew that half of the kids in their class didn't know how to swim. Chapter 5 offers suggestions on how to choose practices most relevant to your situation.

Compassion

Compassion is a sense of concern that arises when we are confronted with pain or suffering and feel motivated to see that suffering relieved.[4] Compassion encompasses awareness, empathy, and action.

Compassion is a natural instinct that everyone has. Some people think of compassion as a feeling or an emotion. Current research suggests that it's more complex and involved. It's more accurate to think of compassion as a skill you can grow and strengthen through practice.

Compassion is a choice, a way of approaching the world, which is why practicing compassion can result in changes in behavior outside of meditation practice.

"Compassion can be viewed as the motive that stimulates and guides us to knowingly notice suffering in self and others, knowingly and empathically connect to make sense and understand the nature and causes of the suffering, and knowingly use empathy and our basic knowledge to search for and implement possible solutions."[5]

PAUL GILBERT & WILLIAM VAN GORDON

Benefits of Mindfulness, Meditation, and Compassion Practices

Mindfulness, meditation, and compassion contribute to a healthy body and healthy mind. The impacts can be small—like feeling a little more calm, relaxed, or focused—or huge—like entering a completely different state of consciousness.

I especially like the way that meditation teacher Jack Kornfield sums up the benefits of practice:

> "Why meditate? Meditative awareness reduces tension and heals the body. Meditation quiets the mind and gently opens the heart. It steadies the spirit. It helps us learn to live more fully in the reality of the present, to see more clearly the people we live with and the world we live in. As we train in mindfulness, we become more present."[6]
>
> **JACK KORNFIELD**

There's a good chance that people who voluntarily join a mindfulness or meditation group will be aware of the benefits and be motivated to participate. However, in a business or classroom setting, it can be helpful to share the positive outcomes of practice with your group to help open their minds to the possibilities and inspire them to participate. Thankfully, there is a mountain of research and data on both the quantitative and qualitative outcomes of mindfulness, meditation, and compassion practices.

For example, these practices have been shown to:

o Lessen depression, anxiety, and stress

o Improve mental clarity and focus

o Increase positive feelings and a sense of connection

Research has revealed a range of specific biological and emotional outcomes:

o Seven minutes of loving-kindness/compassion practice **boosts good feelings, a sense of social connection, and increases relaxation.**[7]

o An eight-week mindfulness class (MBSR) with women with breast cancer measured **beneficial effects on immune function, quality of life, and coping effectiveness.**[8]

o Focused awareness or concentration-based meditation **decreases amygdala activity**—the part of your brain that activates the fight or flight response.[9]

o Self-compassion has been shown to be effective in **reducing both anger and the severity of pain.** It can benefit people in chronic pain even in the absence of other pain management. It can also improve psychological well-being by **decreasing anxiety, depression, and stress** and increasing the capacity to accept pain.[10]

o Benefits of practice happen not just during meditation but **carry over into ordinary life.** Changes in brain function have been measured in beginners who have been practicing for only 8-weeks.[11]

The research can be inspiring, but remember, there is no instant fix. The reason we call it practice is because these are skills that get stronger with repetition over time. The key to unlocking these benefits is helping others work with their awareness—to learn how to draw awareness within and control where they put their attention.

The process of learning to separate awareness from the constant stream of thoughts is both fascinating and subtle. The best evidence of the benefits comes from experiencing it for yourself. Encourage your group to notice how they feel before and after practice. With time, they'll see results for themselves.

Benefits of Group Practice

There are many reasons to do these practices with groups. Here are just a few:

① We are social animals

Having social support can be the determining factor in whether you do something or not. For example, my running buddy kept me jogging every day when I was in college. If she wasn't expecting me, I might have easily skipped.

Just like exercise, we know mindfulness is good for us, but we don't always follow through and do it regularly without some group support. The social aspect of group practice enhances accountability and enriches the experience.

② A friendly guide makes things easier

Say you've just landed in Tokyo, and you don't speak Japanese. As you step off your airplane, you see a smiling face hovering over a sign with your name on it. It's your guide, who will get you to your hotel and make sure you have everything you need for your visit. A supportive guide can help overcome initial barriers, especially for those who are new to the experience and who don't yet "speak the language."

③ We share good vibes

The collective energy of a group can amplify individual experiences, leading to deeper and more meaningful meditative states. My deepest meditations have happened not when I was practicing by myself but when I was sitting in a *group*, in silence, with my eyes closed. How is that different from sitting *alone*, in silence, with my eyes closed?!?

Based on my experience, a group's focus strengthens my individual focus. Some research suggests that it may go even farther than that. For example, a 2012 study found that when a participant was present in the same room with someone meditating on loving-kindness/compassion toward the participant, it directly impacted their physiology—the participant's heart rate slowed and breathing deepened when compared to a control group.[12] That happens in the presence of just one other person—imagine the impact of a room of people sharing good intentions!

④ Presence improves group dynamics

The practices included in this book will engage your group and can change the quality of their attention, their ability to learn new material, to connect with others, and to work together. This benefits each individual and also strengthens the group dynamics as a whole—resulting in groups that are more attentive, cohesive, and collaborative.

Now that you have some foundational information about the what and why of meditation, mindfulness, and compassion practice, it's time to move on to the how. In the next chapter, dive into techniques and tips for successful facilitation. Or, jump to Chapter 4 to learn about the logistics of planning for, and leading, a group.

———

CHAPTER 3

Facilitation Techniques & Tips

This chapter addresses the fundamentals of facilitation that will set you up to be a confident leader, as well as some specific tips for successful facilitation.

If you are an experienced facilitator, you may want to skim this chapter or jump ahead to Chapter 4 to help you prepare for the logistics of your group meeting.

Fundamentals for Facilitators

Grounding yourself in these four cornerstones of facilitation will give you confidence that you can indeed guide a group through a practice—without needing to be perfect.

1. Be compassionate
2. Provide options
3. Treat each person as the expert of their experience
4. Live the practice

1 Be compassionate

There are many ways to be compassionate. For example, you demonstrate compassion by being clear with your instructions, checking in with your group, asking questions, and listening openly to what they share. This includes being compassionate and accepting toward everyone in your group.

While mindfulness, meditation, and compassion practices can be wonderful activities that engage your group and bring great benefit, they can be challenging or uncomfortable for some people. As a facilitator, you set your group up for success by the attitudes you demonstrate when there are questions and discomfort from someone in your group. These are moments when you can apply compassion. Remember that practice in self-awareness brings forth experience that isn't inherently good or bad. It only becomes good or bad when we add a judgment. Your compassionate acceptance sends the message that all experience is welcome and okay.*

---

* Important exceptions are experiences of intense negative feelings that can come up related to trauma and/or PTSD. Read on to the next section for suggestions about how to be compassionate in these situations.

"One compassionate word, action, or thought can reduce another person's suffering and bring them joy. One word can give comfort and confidence, destroy doubt, help someone avoid a mistake, reconcile a conflict, or open the door to liberation. One action can save a person's life or help them take advantage of a rare opportunity. One thought can do the same because thoughts always lead to words and actions. With compassion in our heart, every thought, word, and deed can bring about a miracle."

THICH NHAT HANH

Perhaps the biggest obstacle to successful meditation is the inner critic. We all have an inner critic that is monitoring and judging our actions and sending negative messages like, *"I'm no good at this... Why didn't I...? There's something wrong with me."* It's common for the voice of the inner critic to come up when someone is new to meditation or mindfulness practices—or anything new or unfamiliar for that matter.

Here are some other judgments I've experienced myself or heard from members of my practice groups:

- "I breathe wrong."
- "This is stupid."
- "I'm bad at this."
- "This is boring."
- "My mind is crazy."
- "I can't do this."
- "This is a waste of time."

You can cut the inner critic off at the pass by naming and normalizing these thoughts for your group. Let them know that we all have these thoughts. There's no shame in having them, and there's no need to shut them out. Notice them, *but don't believe them.*

Provide compassionate ways to respond to the inner critic, such as:

- "New things can feel uncomfortable."
- "There's no right or wrong here."
- "Give it some time."
- "Don't give up."
- "Everyone's experience is different, and that's okay."
- "With practice, I can do this."

It's been repeatedly proven through research studies that when you model compassion—toward yourself and others—you help others develop their own skills.

② Provide options

When you imagine someone meditating, what picture comes to mind? Is it someone sitting perfectly still on a cushion, eyes closed, with their legs wrapped up like a pretzel? This image drives many people away from mindfulness practices. I can't tell you how many times I've heard people exclaim, "I have ADHD; there's no way I can meditate." News flash! There are many ways to practice mindfulness and meditation—even with ADHD.

As the leader of your group, be sure you communicate the message that *everyone is different, and that's okay!* The most important thing is that everyone finds an approach that allows them to be comfortable and relaxed.

Give options to the members of your group. Let them know that there's no one-size-fits-all approach. They are the authority of their experience. Give them permission to adjust and adapt based on what makes them comfortable. For example:

- **It's okay to keep your eyes open.** Simply lower and soften your gaze or pick an object in front of you to focus on.

- **It's okay to take a different position.** If sitting is uncomfortable, try lying down or standing up.

- **It's okay to move.** Stretch or rock or even pace back and forth in the room.

- **It's even okay to ignore the meditation instructions.** I like to remind members of my group that they are in the driver's seat. They can think about anything they want, ignore every instruction I give, and (unless they tell me) I won't ever be the wiser. Let people know that if a practice makes them uncomfortable or feel irritated, they don't have to do it! They can change their focus in a way that makes them comfortable, use an anchor (explained below), or do another practice that they know and love.

This kind of guidance is especially important when you consider that an estimated 60% to 70% of all adults have experienced some trauma in their lifetime.[13] Often you will not know what might trigger distress for someone. For example, in her book *It's OK That You're Not OK*, psychologist Megan Divine tells of her experience and grief at the sudden drowning death of her husband. Pretty much every mindfulness practice includes instructions to connect to the breath. Many practices, including ones in this book, focus on the breath entirely. But for Megan, focusing on the breath only triggered thoughts of her husband's death. This may seem like an extreme example, but you never know where someone may be coming from. Check in with people and give them options to choose something that feels safe.

Another example of a "typical" instruction that can be uncomfortable for some people is closing the eyes. It can be hard for someone to feel safe with their eyes closed in a room full of people they do not know well. It's fine to just look down or away and not close the eyes. Again, offer variations and repeat, and repeat again, that each person should choose what's right for them.

Many people also respond negatively to orders or commands. Mushim Patricia Ikeda from the East Bay Meditation Center explains their approach to keeping instructions inclusive in this way:

"Instead of using a language of 'command,' we use invitational language. We give people a lot of choices within the parameters of meditation techniques. We use invitations such as 'If this is accessible to you,' 'If this is available to you,' 'If you like,' 'You might try both and see what makes you feel safer.'"[14]

MUSHIM PATRICIA IKEDA

USING AN ANCHOR

An anchor is a useful concept to introduce to your group. It's a tool used in meditation that can create a sense of safety and comfort. An anchor is anything that connects you to the present moment—like feeling the soles of your feet in contact with the floor or focusing on the sensations in your hands. Other possible anchors include focusing on the breath or repeating a mantra. Some people keep a special coin or stone in their pocket to touch as a reminder to pause and bring awareness to the present.

Just as the word suggests, during meditation, an anchor can keep you from going adrift. When you get swept away by thoughts or emotions, or feel lost in a practice, you can always bring your focus back to the anchor.

Everyone has wandering thoughts, so an anchor is useful for anyone, but an anchor is especially helpful for those who experience difficult emotions. Sometimes people can feel distressed during a meditation, whether they are confronted with a difficult memory or with harsh internal judgments or self-criticism. Remembering and using an anchor can be a lifeline back to a feeling of safety and security in the present moment.

If you have an ongoing group, you might encourage members to find an anchor that works for them and use it during practice sessions when they need something safe to focus on.

MORE USES FOR AN ANCHOR

An anchor is also a useful tool to help redirect thoughts outside of meditation, because ultimately our goal is to be mindful not just when we close our eyes but throughout our day.

You can use an anchor whenever you are feeling angry, anxious, unsettled, or overwhelmed—or anytime you want to feel more stability and connection to the present moment.

Connecting to an anchor can be done in a few minutes or seconds—pretty much anywhere, anytime.

③ Treat each person as the expert of their experience

It's your job as a facilitator to create conditions for each member of your group to discover their own inner experience. You can't have the experience for them. You can lead them to the door of the castle, but you can't go inside. You can only wait for them to come back and report what they found.

When they do, be curious, kind, and nonjudgmental about anything they report. There's no right or wrong, good or bad. Everyone's experience is unique and that's interesting! People recognize when they are being accepted wholeheartedly. It makes them feel valued and respected. When you accept their experience as it is, you support their process of self-awareness. That's where the gold lies.

Here's an example of how this might show up. Recently I was leading Inside Outside (Practice 2.4). One step of this practice is to sense the space inside your body. Then, shift focus and see if you can sense the space around you, outside of your body. After the practice finished, one of the group members reported that she didn't like it. She was comfortable and calm sensing inside her body but sensing beyond that, "just didn't feel good."

As she spoke, I thought to myself, "*Oh no! It's so cool to try to extend your sensory perception into the space around you.*" But my job wasn't to convince her why "outside" was good. When someone shares their experience, don't argue with them! You don't need to change them. Be curious and let them know that whatever they experience, it's okay and interesting and worthwhile. So, I kept my thoughts to myself and said, "That's so interesting. Now you know that focusing on internal sensations feels good. It's okay to stick with that. If something feels wrong for you, you don't have to do it."

Another challenge you may face is people who either report having no reaction at all or say they are not "getting it." For example, in Practice 5.1 Loving-Kindness, the instructions include "notice any positive thoughts, feelings of gratitude, affection, or warmth," however not everyone feels warm, and sometimes people will report that they "didn't feel any-thing." Accept that and validate that. "It's okay. It's enough to simply practice. Just because you don't pick up on a physical sensation doesn't mean that your efforts in loving-kindness aren't working. Everyone experiences this practice in a dif-ferent way."

On a practical level, you can show respect and acceptance for each person by applying active listening skills. Active listen-ing means listening with the intent to really understand. An important component of active listening is repeating back or paraphrasing what's been said.* In the example above, I might start by saying, "So, you didn't notice any physical changes during the practice?" Then, give an opportunity for the person to confirm, clarify, or elaborate. Reflecting back what a person says shows them that their experience is important and gives them a chance to gain more self-awareness.

④ Live the practice

As you facilitate practices, you'll have ongoing opportunities to develop your skills. Holding space for others requires active participation. You can talk about being present, aware, open, nonjudgmental, and compassionate, but how can you expect others to embrace these states if you don't do it yourself?

---

* Other components of active listening include asking open-ended questions, using positive body language and eye contact, and being affirmative and encourag-ing. Active listen skills will help you be a great facilitator. Find out more in the Resources section at the end of this book.

To embody something is to represent it in bodily form. It requires getting out of your head. One way to do that is to pay attention to the physical sensations in your body. What physical sensations do you experience when you practice meditation, mindfulness, and compassion? Perhaps your shoulders or face are more relaxed. Maybe you feel warmth in your chest or belly, or parts of your body feel energized. Ideally, you'll be in this state when leading a meditation as well.

At first, facilitating a practice may make you feel self-conscious or may require a lot of thinking, making it difficult to live the practice in the moment. That's normal. As you gain experience, you will be able to both embody the practice *and* facilitate.

A final way you can embody the practice is by remembering that it doesn't have to be serious. No one is perfect—not even you! Mindfulness includes curiosity, humor, playfulness, and joy. Being authentic and sharing your experiences will help members of your group feel safe sharing theirs—creating a virtuous cycle of learning.

Facilitation Tips

Sharing and Discussion

When including a short mindfulness practice as part of a larger meeting or class, you may or may not choose to include a group discussion or dialog about the experience. But for a more regular group with extended time to practice, you will most likely want to encourage people to share their experience after a practice.

Allowing time for members to reflect is a great way to culti-vate engagement, deeper learning, and a sense of common humanity within your group. (*"What?!? I'm not the only one with a wandering mind?"*) And it emphasizes how important it is to learn from personal experience.

Whatever your setting, when you want to encourage discus-sion and sharing, let people know in advance that they'll have this opportunity. Then, when you open the floor, be curious and interested.

With a larger group, you can get everyone engaged by asking for a show of hands in response to a prompt:

- "How many of you noticed your mind was very busy today?"
- "How many of you feel calmer now than before? Yes? No?"

Then try some conversation starters for individual sharing:

- "How did that go for you?"
- "What did you notice about that practice?"
- "When your mind wandered, where did it go?"

Use active listening and paraphrase what you hear someone say to let them know they were understood. Include a follow-up question (like, "Did I get that right?"), and allow space for them to clarify or add more. Remember to take on the role of a kind and inquisitive interviewer. Your acceptance and attention will create space for collaborative learning.

Managing Group Dynamics

When facilitating group discussion, part of your job will be to keep things on track. You want to allow group participation and encourage sharing that's on topic and balanced among the group's members. Be aware of when things start to go off track. For example, if you have one or two people doing most of the talking, you may need to jump in, acknowledge what they've said, and then open up the discussion by inviting others to share.

Here are some ways to bring others into a conversation:

- "Did anyone else experience what Sam is describing?"
- "Let's pause for a moment. I want to make sure that everyone who wants to share has an opportunity to do that."

Facilitating groups effectively is like a beautiful dance of give and take. The guidelines above represent only the tip of the iceberg. Your skill as a group facilitator will develop with time and practice. Start to notice the dynamics in other groups you participate in, learn from other leaders, and apply that knowledge to your own situation.

"A teacher's authority is not hierarchical. It is grounded in a clear sense of being thoroughly 'at home' within this process of learning and of knowing this process well because [they have] trodden this path, too."[15]

MANUAL OF THE MINDFULNESS-BASED INTERVENTIONS TEACHING ASSESSMENT CRITERIA

REFLECT

Are you clear about what you want to bring to your group as a facilitator? You can use mindfulness to set your intentions, attention, and attitude before leading a group. See below for some examples and take a moment to record your goals in these areas.

Intention

Create a space for healing, creativity, peace...

Attention

Focused, present, calm....

Attitude

Open, curious, kind, accepting...

Continue to Chapter 4 for specific recommendations on how to plan for, and lead, a practice group.

CHAPTER 4

Logistics

This chapter addresses the nuts and bolts of facilitating groups through mindfulness, meditation, and compassion practices, including:

o What to do in advance of your group meeting to make sure things go smoothly

o Detailed instructions for opening and closing any practice

If you are an experienced teacher or facilitator, you may want to skim this chapter or jump ahead to Chapter 5 to explore the practices. If you are just getting started, here's a kind of preflight checklist to help you prepare.

Meeting Logistics

In-Person Meetings

Your physical space is equally important to setting the tone for your group as your presentation and tone of voice. Some suggestions include:

o Arrange the chairs in a circle.

o Remove clutter.

o Silence your phone and/or devices and ask your group members to do the same.

o Don't play music. Some people recommend playing ambient music during practice. I emphatically do not. If your goal is to allow people to connect with their inner experience, music is more likely to distract than to assist in this process.

o Remove distractions from the room—like a clock with a loud tick or a vase of flowers with a strong scent.

Sometimes there will be aspects of your meeting space that are outside your control, like traffic going by or a noisy heating system. You can reassure your group that distractions are just another opportunity to practice. When you notice the distraction and return focus to your practice, it strengthens your mindfulness skills.

Online Meetings

Setting up your space is equally important for groups that meet virtually:

- Ask members to turn on their video and select a view that allows them to see everyone attending. This will strengthen the connection of the group.

- Sit in a place with good light and without clutter in the background, or use a background filter, so that everyone can see you well.

- Ask people to mute themselves during practices to avoid distractions for others in the group.

Some people feel self-conscious leaving the camera on when they close their eyes for a practice. Let people know that it's okay to turn off their camera during a practice, if it makes them more comfortable, and ask them to turn their camera back on after the practice is over and you are returning to group discussion.

Format

The practices outlined in the next chapter can be adapted to work within different timeframes. If you are planning to use a practice as a simple five- to 10-minute centering exercise for your group before a meeting, workshop, or class, your format will be straightforward. Follow the instructions for opening and closing a practice below, and when you're done, carry on with your agenda for your group.

If you are planning for a 30- to 60-minute practice as part of a workplace stress reduction program or in a healthcare setting, then it can be helpful to formalize a format for your group. As an example, my regular mindful meditation circle meets for an hour. During that time, we include three rounds of meditation of about seven to 12 minutes each. We also allow time for group members to check in, reflect, and ask questions.

The first round of meditation is always a breath- or body-based meditation with the goal of allowing members to arrive, center, settle, calm the mind, and relax. The third round of meditation is always a compassion meditation, so that we close with a feeling of connection and community. In between, we stay open to whatever theme or interest arises from the group or the facilitator. A complete template of this kind of group format is included at the end of the Resources section.

For each round of practice, I find that five to 12 minutes is a good length for people who have little experience with meditation. For those with more experience, 15 to 30 minutes may be comfortable. Experiment and ask your group what feels right. When in doubt, start small. It's better for a practice to be too short and have people wishing for more, than to go too long, leaving people feeling uncomfortable, impatient, or lost.

To help yourself keep track of time, you can use a timer. This allows you to focus on the practice and not need to stop and look at a clock. Most phones have a gentle ringtone of chimes or birdsong. Tell your group, "We're going to do this for about eight minutes. I'm going to set a timer. When you hear it go off, I'll start to wrap up the practice."

Agreements

Group agreements set parameters for discussion and interaction. Depending on your group, it may be helpful to set expectations upfront about attendance, timeliness, confidentiality, not interrupting each other, or any other aspect of group behavior. Think about the kind of group dynamics you'd like and tailor your agreements accordingly.

As an example, here are agreements used by Healing Circles Global[16] that are simple and provide guidance for how the group will engage:

- We treat each other with kindness and respect.
- We listen with compassion and curiosity.
- We honor each other's unique experiences and don't presume to advise, fix, or save one other.
- What we share in circle is confidential.
- We trust each of us has guidance we need within us, and we rely on the power of silence to access it.

It's inevitable that at some point someone in your group will give unsolicited advice. Giving advice can be a knee-jerk habit for many people. After all, we're well-meaning people and we want to help others.

Including a statement such as "we don't presume to advise or fix" as part of your group agreements can help you redirect gracefully and without adding shame. When someone starts giving advice, you can say, "Remember our group agreement. We're here to listen, not to give advice." I also reassure people that it's natural to want to offer suggestions. Encourage people to notice the urge to give advice. It's an act of mindfulness to notice that urge but instead stay silent, listen, and allow others space to process their thoughts.

Prepare Yourself

Practice

In the theater world, before you present a play or musical to an audience, you first do a dress-rehearsal (or two or three) to work out any rough spots. Why? Because no one, not even you, makes a perfect delivery without some practice. As a beginning facilitator, it's helpful to sit in a room by yourself, turn on a recording device, and try talking through a practice. Then, listen back to your recording—remembering to be kind and self-compassionate. Notice any moments where things were rushed, or perhaps a little bumpy.

Here's an example of something I discovered when I started recording and listening back to myself. In my attempt to slow down and create space, I sometimes paused in the middle of a thought or sentence. It's distracting when...

...

...you are left hanging with half the message. (*See what I mean?!?*) By listening back to myself, I've learned to be conscious of completing my sentences before pausing.

Pacing

Which brings us to the topic of pacing. When facilitating a practice, you create space for your group to slow down and have an internal experience. This means you need to allow time for silence. When you relax and slow down, your group can relax and slow down too. Embrace the pause, breathe, and experiment to find a pace that feels comfortable.

Of course there's no perfect pace for your guided meditation. Some people will prefer hearing regular guidance, while others like more space and silence. You know the saying: you can't please all of the people all of the time. Still, there are things you can do to ensure that your delivery style works for a majority of people.

In general, beginners appreciate regular guidance, while those with more experience may prefer longer stretches of silence. You can measure your pauses by counting the breath. Take two to five deep breaths for a short pause and up to 10 or more breaths for a longer pause. When I first started, I kept a timer by my side so I could gauge my pace. With practice, I've developed my sense of time so that I no longer need to rely on a timer, and you probably will too.

If you plan to spend several minutes in silence, let the group know. For example, "We'll spend three or four minutes in silence." Then, when you begin again after a period of silence, be gentle and allow time for people to transition back. "Begin to bring your awareness back..." or "Before we bring the practice to a close..."

Tone of Voice

Listening to your own voice, especially when listening back to a recording, makes many people self-conscious. Don't fret over your voice too much. Instead, focus on the qualities you want to evoke—kindness, calm, alertness, openness—and embody them. Bring to mind the kind of space that you want to create for your group and trust that this will come through in your voice.

Don't believe me? Back when I worked in business and sales, some common advice was to smile before answering the telephone. Why? Because you can make your tone of voice more friendly simply by the act of smiling. You can try this out by recording yourself. Say something, and then consciously smile and say it again. I bet you'll find the second version warmer and more welcoming.

Volume

Be aware of the volume of your voice. It's not relaxing to have to strain to hear someone speak. Articulate your words clearly and speak at a volume that can be easily heard throughout the room. Of course, you don't want to shout either. Be sensitive to members of your group who have hearing difficulties and use a microphone or encourage them to sit toward the front of the room if needed.

Preparation Checklist

Are you ready?
Here's a checklist to help you prepare.

SEVERAL WEEKS BEFORE

☐ Decide on the purpose and format of the group.

☐ Consider any group agreements you'd like to have.

☐ Choose the meeting place and time.

☐ Invite people to the group.

A DAY OR TWO BEFORE

☐ Create an outline for how you will use your time.

☐ Choose the practices you will facilitate.

☐ Practice how you will introduce and lead the practices.

☐ Gather materials, like a timer or any handouts you will share.

THE DAY OF

☐ Prepare the space (either physical or virtual).

☐ Believe in yourself!

Orienting the Group

Safety Instructions

You create a comfortable and positive experience for your group through your words and actions. Just as an airline attendant's job is to review the safety instructions before every flight, your job is to ensure that everyone participating in a practice gets to their destination safely—including knowing what to do in the event of an emergency.

Especially when working with beginners or any new group, "safety instructions" include explaining practical details before you start each session. People can be more relaxed when they know what to expect. Here are common questions that are helpful to anticipate and address:

① Why are we doing this?

It may be obvious to you that group practice is going to help everyone be more focused or calm or creative or connected. But the purpose may be less clear for someone who hasn't experienced it before. Be sure to share the reason(s) for your practice. By sharing your intention, you help create positive intentions within your group.

② How long will it take?

As you orient your group, let them know about how long the practice will last. Otherwise, sitting through a guided practice can feel like being a kid stuck on a long car ride. ("How much longer is this going to take? I need to go to the bathroom!")

③ How to sit (or lie down, or stand)?

The best position to take during any practice is one that allows you to be comfortable and alert. In general, sitting upright is a good posture to take. "Sit upright with your feet firmly on the floor." For some people, however, sitting may not be comfortable. Before you begin, let people know that it's okay to adapt and do whatever they need to do to be comfortable. This could include sitting on the floor on a firm pillow, lying on the ground with knees bent and the soles of the feet on the floor, or standing with a hand on a chair or wall.

④ Where to look?

With all but a few exceptions, the practices described here involve focusing awareness internally. To support this, while also giving people options, you can instruct people to either close their eyes, or lower their gaze—keeping a soft focus in front of them.

⑤ How to breathe?

For all practices, breathing should be easy and comfortable and done in and out through the nose—unless you are congested or otherwise unable to breathe through your nose.

Once you've addressed common questions, you can begin leading your practice(s).

Opening and Closing

No matter what practice you are leading, you'll begin with instructions to help people get settled and end with some words to bring closure. The practices outlined in Chapter 5 include abbreviated opening and closing instructions. Below, you'll find detailed scripts for leading a group into, and out of, a practice successfully. These can be used as a container for any practice in Chapter 5. They can also be expanded and used as a mini-mindfulness exercise all on their own. Especially in a business setting when you have only 5 minutes, settling a group's attention through one of the five awareness practices below may be all that you need.

An opening can take anywhere from one to 10 minutes, depending on the time you have available for your practice. Take time between each step to pause and give people space and permission to slow down. You can adjust the length of your pauses depending on the amount of time you have.

A closing provides time and space for members of your group to transition from a state of inner focus to a state of reengagement with the external world. You may allow several minutes for people to "come back" after a longer practice, or something as brief as 30 seconds to close out a shorter practice.

You'll notice that these instructions include some combination of bringing attention to the present moment through awareness of the environment, body, breath, and/or mind. A wise teacher of mine recommends that, as a guide, it's helpful to "back out the same way you got in." So whatever focus you choose as your opening, return to this anchor as you close.

The opening and closing scripts are paired, so you can see how they work together.

Variations for Opening and Closing

The next pages include several variations for opening and closing guided practices. Use and adapt these so that they feel natural to you.

AWARENESS OF BODY AND BREATH

OPENING SCRIPT

"Find a comfortable position, either seated or lying down..." *Pause.*

"You can close your eyes or lower your gaze and begin to draw your awareness within..." *Pause.*

"Notice and adjust your posture so you are comfortable and supported..." *Pause.*

"Rest and relax your hands in your lap or at your sides..." *Pause.*

"Relax your shoulders... neck... jaw... and face..." *Pause.*

"Set aside any thoughts as you turn your awareness to the breath..." *Pause.*

"There's no need to change your breathing, just watch it happen however it's happening..." *Pause.*

"Allowing yourself to arrive here, in the present moment."

CLOSING SCRIPT

"...As we begin to bring this practice to a close, rest your attention on the breath, noticing the air coming in and going out." *Pause.*

"...Then shift your attention to the body. Notice points of contact... maybe feel your feet flat on the ground, or your hands resting on your lap." *Pause.*

"...When you're ready, you can open your eyes." *Pause.*

"...Thank you."

AWARENESS OF BODY

OPENING SCRIPT

"Sit in a comfortable position and close the eyes or soften your gaze..." *Pause.*

"Breathing slowly through your nose, notice the sensations you can feel in your body—knowing that whatever you experience is okay just as it is..." *Pause.*

"Feel the places where your body is in contact with the floor or chair. Feel any sensations in the bottoms of your feet. Notice the pressure in your seat as gravity roots you to the ground, pulling you to the earth..." *Pause.*

"Adjust your posture so you feel centered. Allow your spine to lengthen and feel the top of the head rising toward the sky..." *Pause.*

"Notice both feelings together. Drawing down to the ground and rising up toward the sky."

CLOSING SCRIPT

"...In a moment, we're going to come back." *Pause.*

"...Become aware of the contact of your body with the chair, and the floor—and by extension your contact with the earth." *Pause.*

"...For a moment feel the massiveness of the earth and the effects of its gravity holding you to the floor." *Pause.*

"...Maybe wiggle your toes, your fingers." *Pause.*

"...And when you are ready, let the eyes open."

AWARENESS OF BREATH

___

OPENING SCRIPT

___

"Start by drawing your awareness within. Close your eyes or gently gaze down toward the floor..." *Pause.*

"Bring your awareness to how you are sitting (or standing or lying down). *Pause.*

"Scan the body. Notice any tension and adjust your body to get comfortable..." *Pause.*

"Begin by taking two or three deep breaths—inhaling through the nose and exhaling through the mouth, making a "ha" or sighing sound..." *Pause.*

"Then allow your breathing to settle into its own rhythm, breathing in *and out* through the nose..." *Pause.*

"For a few moments, just focus on your breath. Let yourself experience and be aware of the sensations of breathing. Do you feel the belly going in and out... the rib cage expanding and relaxing... the air as it passes through the nostrils or the throat?..." *Pause.*

"Take a moment to rest in the breath."

___

CLOSING SCRIPT

"...In the last few moments, simply allow your body and mind to rest in the natural rhythm of your breath." *Pause.*

"...Feel the whole body breathing." *Pause.*

"...And when you are ready, let the eyes open."

AWARENESS OF THOUGHTS

OPENING SCRIPT

"Sitting comfortably, relax the face and shoulders..."
Pause.

"You may want to close your eyes or lower your gaze..."
Pause.

"Take a moment to observe what's going on inside..."
Pause.

"Notice any thoughts or feelings... Notice sensations in your body... What's going on inside you right now?..."
Pause.

"Allow things to be just as they are..." *Pause.*

"For this practice, set an intention to be open, curious, and kind to yourself."

CLOSING SCRIPT

"...As we draw this practice to a close, notice any effects this practice has had on your state of mind and body." *Pause.*

"...When you are ready, gently open your eyes and return to the room."

AWARENESS OF YOUR SURROUNDINGS

As noted in Chapter 3, for a variety of reasons, connecting with the body or breath may be uncomfortable for some people. A colleague of mine, who works with individuals who have experienced trauma, recommends focusing on the external environment as an opening for practice.[17]

OPENING SCRIPT

"As you sit, begin to notice the details of this moment and place..." *Pause.*

"Notice the temperature of this room... the color of the walls..." *Pause.*

"Lower your gaze or perhaps close the eyes. What sounds do you hear? Are they near or far?..." *Pause.*

"Next, see if you can feel the bottoms of your feet as they rest on the floor..." *Pause.*

"Notice what you are feeling right now. It may be boredom, resistance, sleepiness, restlessness, quiet. Allow yourself to simply be as you are in this moment."

CLOSING SCRIPT

"...As we draw this practice to a close, start to shift your awareness back to the room around you." *Pause.*

"...Notice any sounds. Notice the feeling of the air on your skin." *Pause.*

"...Can you sense the shape of the room and the walls around you?" *Pause.*

"...When you are ready, you can open your eyes and again notice the details of the room." *Pause.*

"...Thank you."

PHYSIOLOGICAL SIGH

The Breath Awareness script includes instructions to inhale through the nose and exhale through an open mouth while making a "ha" or sighing sound. This kind of sigh has been shown in research studies to be a quick and effective way to calm the body. Extended exhalation slows down the heart rate and has an overall soothing effect on the body.

If you want to get really geeky about it, you can share the "gold standard" practice called the physiological sigh. The physiological sigh is based on a pattern of breathing that can happen involuntarily when carbon dioxide builds up in the bloodstream and triggers the impulse to breathe. The pattern is *two* inhales through the nose followed by a long exhale through the mouth. The second inhale helps inflate the air sacs in the lungs to improve the release of carbon dioxide from the blood. Here's a good way to describe the process:

"Breathe in through your nose. When you've comfortably filled your lungs, take a second, deeper sip of air to expand your lungs as much as possible. Then, very slowly, exhale through your mouth until all the air is gone."

Researchers at Stanford University have found this controlled-breathing practice reduces stress. People who did five minutes of this breathing every day reported significant improvement in mood, and with regular practice, experienced a slower breathing rate overall throughout the day.[18]

OPENING WITH INTENTIONS AND CLOSING WITH AFFIRMATIONS

Both intentions and affirmations can amplify the positive effects of meditation, mindfulness, and compassion practices.

If you are inclined, guiding people to set their intention for practice fits nicely during the introduction or opening. Saying something like, "Take a moment to connect with your intentions for this practice," can help people find their own intrinsic motivation.

Affirmations can be added at the close of a practice. I love the closing used in the YoMind video series, Mindful Moments with JusTme.[9] This program is designed for kids, but I find it works great with adults who want to connect with their inner child. It goes like this:

"Repeat after me, either in a whisper or in your head... It's okay to be awesome. I *am* awesome. It's okay to be great. I *am* great. When I work hard and set my mind to it, I can do it. I can be my best, and I can do my best, because I *am* my best.

Inhale the arms up and take a full-body stretch. Bring the arms back down and relax. Excellent job!"

Now that you have ideas for opening and closing a practice, it's time to explore a range of practices you can use. Chapter 5 gives you 27 practices to choose from, as well as suggestions on how to pick the best practices for your group.

———

CHAPTER 5

Practices

In this chapter, you'll find 27 meditation and mindfulness practices organized into five categories:

(**1**) Breath-based practices

(**2**) Body-based practices

(**3**) Focused awareness practices

(**4**) Open awareness practices

(**5**) Compassion practices

You'll also find advice and reference charts to help you identify how to choose practices that suit you and your group.

As the categories suggest, the practices address a range of desired outcomes—such as physical relaxation, greater self-compassion, and increased mental clarity. Each one includes an outline with specific instructions to read out loud. There are also tips and suggested variations that you can choose to use, or not, depending on your situation.

Once you are familiar with the content and the shape of each practice, feel free to expand or modify the script. Remember to add time for space and silence. Experiment and you will discover how to make these your own.

The openings and closings are brief, so look to Chapter 4 for in-depth guidance on how to begin and end a practice, including a handful of more detailed scripts that you can use in tandem with any of the practices in this chapter.

How to Choose Practices

As you know, this book is designed to make leading group practices easy and doable for everyone. You don't need to be an expert in every possible method to start facilitating. Here are some guidelines on how to choose which practices to use.

① Pick practices that you feel comfortable with

Chances are, you are holding this book because you've had some experience with mindfulness or meditation practices. What have you found helpful? Scan the options here and identify the ones that you have personal experience with and an authentic connection to. Start in your comfort zone. The more comfortable you feel with the practice, the more confidently you'll be able to describe and guide the practice. That ease and familiarity will make for a positive experience for your group.

② Match practices to your group's experience level and dynamics

When choosing practices, the age and level of experience of your group will influence your choices. For example, if you are working with beginners, it's helpful to start with something that is very specific and clear—like counting or focusing on the breath. With kids, something that's tangible helps hold their attention. Finger tracing is one of my favorites to do with kids.

If you have a group with mixed experience levels, focus on the newbies. Slow down and ensure your instructions are clear and all their questions are answered before starting. Even someone with experience will appreciate your efforts to be inclusive and will find value in "basic" practices.

Finally, consider your group's dynamics. Are the members comfortable sharing personal and potentially emotional experiences? Or are you working with a new group or in a more formal setting? No matter who is in your group, you want everyone to feel safe. Breath-based practices and focused awareness practices tend to be more neutral in content and can be a safe place to start.

SUGGESTED PRACTICES BASED ON GROUP CHARACTERISTICS

Kids	1.3.	Finger Tracing
	1.6.	Coherent Breathing
	4.1.	Awareness of Your Environment
	5.2.	Find a Compassionate Image
	5.6.	Just Like Me
Beginners	1.1.	Mindfulness of Breathing
	1.2.	The Zen 10
	4.1.	Awareness of Your Environment
	4.4.	Mindful Listening
	5.2.	Find a Compassionate Image
People with experience	1.5.	Slowing Down the Exhale (aka 4:2:6)
	1.7.	Watching the Cycles of Breathing
	4.2.	Observing Thoughts
	5.4.	Self-Compassion
Groups whose members are comfortable with each other	2.0.	Body-Based Practices
	5.0.	Compassion Practices
Groups whose members are less familiar with each other	1.0.	Breath-Based Practices
	3.0.	Focused Awareness Practices

③ Match practices to the benefits you are seeking

Significant research has been conducted in the past decades on the measurable outcomes of the practices included in this guidebook. Through a range of studies that includes brain scans, attention and stress testing, and self-reporting, we know that different practices have different effects,[20, 21] including:

o Improved concentration

o Increased feelings of connection, joy, gratitude, and hope

o Increased ability to manage emotions and anxiety

o Increased ability to cope with social stress

There is some overlap. For example, both mindfulness and compassion meditation improve attention and focus. However, there are also distinct differences. Below are some suggested practices organized according to Dr. Kelly McGonigal's framework for the benefits of meditation on attention, compassion/connection, and stress reduction.[22]

SUGGESTED PRACTICES BASED ON DESIRED OUTCOME

Improve Attention

Distracted → Focused	1.2. The Zen 10
	3.1. Using a Mantra
	3.3. Counting Backward
Frenetic → Centered	1.2. The Zen 10
	1.4. Belly Breathing
	1.6. Coherent Breathing
	3.2. Gazing
Fixated → Open/Creative	2.4. Inside Outside
	4.2. Observing Thoughts
	5.1. Loving-Kindness

Increase Compassion

Disconnected → Connected	4.4. Mindful Listening
	5.1. Loving-Kindness
	5.3. Compassion for a Loved One
	5.7. Tonglen

Reduce Stress

Anxious → Calm	1.1. Mindfulness of Breathing
	1.4. Belly Breathing
	2.1. Body Scan
	4.3. Name It to Tame It
Tense → Relaxed	1.1. Mindfulness of Breathing
	1.5. Slowing Down the Exhale (aka 4:2:6)
	2.1. Body Scan
	2.2. Working with Physical Pain
	5.2. Find a Compassionate Image
Distressed → Grounded	1.3. Finger Tracing
	2.3. Walking Meditation
	2.6 Grounded Like a Tree
	4.1. Awareness of Your Environment
	4.3. Name It to Tame It
	5.5. Compassionate Touch

④ Choose practices connected to your group's purpose or theme

Your group's purpose or theme may guide you to relevant practices. For example, if your work team wants to do a three-minute centering practice before a planning meeting, your choices may be different than if you are leading a guided meditation at the end of a yoga class. The suggestions below are merely a starting place to use as you explore what is appropriate for your group.

SUGGESTED PRACTICES BASED ON GROUP THEMES

Arriving/Centering

- 1.6. Coherent Breathing
- 2.5. Cloud Hands
- 4.1. Awareness of Your Environment
- 4.4. Mindful Listening
- 5.6. Just Like Me

Mindfulness

- 4.0. Open Awareness Practices
- 1.0. Breath-Based Practices
- 2.0. Body-Based Practices

Self-Discovery

- 1.1. Mindfulness of Breathing
- 2.2. Working with Physical Pain
- 4.2. Observing Thoughts
- 5.2. Find a Compassionate Image
- 5.4. Self-Compassion

Health and Wellness

1.4. Belly Breathing

1.5. Slowing Down the Exhale (aka 4:2:6)

2.1. Body Scan

2.2. Working with Physical Pain

4.3. Name It to Tame It

5.2. Find a Compassionate Image

5.4. Self-Compassion

5.5. Compassionate Touch

5.6. Just Like Me

Spirituality

5.0. Compassion Practices

Section 1:
Breath-Based Practices

To say that breathing is good for us, is obvious. But did you know that five to 10 minutes of deep breathing can stimulate the immune system, lower blood pressure, and increase energy levels? Breathing practices are good for stress reduction and for cultivating awareness and focus.

The breath is a unique entry point for centering and mindfulness, because it is the one involuntary bodily function that everyone can easily control. By contrast, can you consciously choose to stop digesting the food in your stomach, lower your blood pressure on command, or quiet those crazy thoughts in the middle of the night? For most people, the answer is no. But I bet if I asked you to hold your breath for five seconds, you could take control and do this easily.

Breathing practices have been developed and used for centuries to support both mental and physical health and to reach different states of consciousness. They can serve as a shortcut to quiet the mind. In the yoga tradition, breath practice is used as a preparation for meditation because it is calming and it supports concentration—steadying the mind and improving mental clarity.

"The mind can go in many directions in a split second. Its movements are very fast and varied. But the breath cannot go in many directions at once. It has only one path: inhalation and exhalation. It can pause for a moment in a state of retention, but it cannot multiply like the mind. ... Controlling the breath and observing its rhythm brings the consciousness to stillness. ... By controlling the breath, you are controlling consciousness, and by controlling consciousness, you bring rhythm to the breath."

B.K.S. IYENGAR, *THE TREE OF YOGA*

———————

Changing our breath can change our physiology and our state of mind because the nervous system and respiratory system are closely linked. There's a reason why people say, "take a deep breath," when you are upset or angry. We can use the breath to help us calm down.

Breath-based practices are great for these reasons and more. They are direct and effective, and they work well for beginners and more experienced meditators.

1.1. MINDFULNESS OF BREATHING

Good for:

- Beginners
- Calming down
- Reducing stress

Introduction

Perhaps the most foundational meditation practice is mindfulness of breathing. One reason for this is that the breath is always with you, now, in the present moment.

The practice is done exactly as you would imagine, focusing on the breath and sensations of breathing with alertness, curiosity, and kindness.

How to Practice

- Find a comfortable seated position.

- Draw the awareness within. Notice and adjust your posture. Rest and relax your hands in the lap.

- Set aside any thoughts as you turn your awareness to the breath.

- There's no need to change your breathing, just watch it happen however it's happening.

- You might start by labeling the breath—silently saying to yourself "inhale/exhale," or "in/out," as you breathe.

- Or use these phrases from Thich Nhat Hanh, "Breathing in, I know I am breathing in. Breathing out, I know I am breathing out."

- Be a curious observer and notice when something else comes into the mind—a judgment, a memory, a plan, an emotion. When you notice that happen, celebrate the fact that you noticed it! It's normal for thoughts to come up. When they do, it's an opportunity to practice letting go of the thought and, gently and kindly, to return focus back to labeling the breath.

Variation

For some people, labeling each inhalation and exhalation creates a steady focus. For others, it is easier to maintain focus on the *sensations* of breathing.

o Bring awareness to the breath.

o Notice where you feel the sensations of breathing in the body. For example, you might feel the air flowing in and out of the nostrils, or the rising and falling of the belly, or expansion and relaxation of the chest.

o Be a curious observer and notice the details of these sensations as they happen and how they may change over time.

Tips

o Experiment with both labeling the breath and focusing on the sensations of breathing to see which one feels more natural to you.

o To help calm and steady the mind, give your brain permission to rest. Think of resting the mind on the breath as if resting on a big feather cushion. Or imagine that you're standing in a stream of thoughts and that you can step out of the stream and rest on the bank. The stream of thoughts may continue, but you can take a break from it.

o When you stop and notice each thought that comes up, you will gain a new level of self-awareness. I am continually astonished by how nonlinear my brain is and how my thoughts jump around through a series of sometimes obvious, sometimes comical, and sometimes mysterious associations. Taking the perspective of a curious observer of your own mind can be hugely entertaining and enlightening.

WHAT TO DO WITH A RACING MIND

Perhaps the most common challenge people face in meditation is learning how to work with an active mind. You may begin following the instructions and then realize that your mind has wandered and you're thinking of something else.

First and foremost, know that thinking is normal. I like to tell people, "You wouldn't want your heart to stop beating or your lungs to stop breathing, would you? The heart is going to beat, the lungs are going to breathe, and the brain is going to generate thoughts." Yet there is more to your consciousness than the thoughts that pass through your head. With meditation and mindfulness practices, we consciously shift focus away from thinking toward an alert and open awareness. And we do it over, and over, and over, and over, and over (you get my point) again.

You may arrive at a place in this practice where you feel frustrated by the noise of all the thoughts and wonder, "What's the point of this anyway?!" Or you might decide that meditation is not for you, or that you can't do meditation. Don't give up! Having thoughts and noticing those thoughts are part of the process.

With practice, you will learn how to steady and calm busy thoughts. Keep going and you will develop the ability to connect to a larger awareness and find a centered sense of peace, happiness, health, and healing. It may last for only a few minutes or a few seconds at first, but ultimately you are hardwiring your brain with this valuable way of being.

Something that helps me be kind to my active mind is to imagine my thoughts as little children. I pretend I'm a teacher sitting at the head of a circle in a kindergarten class. When thoughts jump up, like young children that have trouble sitting still, I imagine patting them on the head in a kind way and saying something like, "Settle down. We're going to sit still for a little while. When we're done, you can go outside and play."

1.2. THE ZEN 10

Good for:

- Beginners
- Increasing focus/concentration
- Quieting a busy mind

Introduction

The Zen 10 meditation is a breath-based meditation that comes from the Zen Buddhist tradition. It's a great practice, especially for beginners, because it is so straightforward. If you are breathing and you can count to 10, then you can do this one.

You can practice this meditation sitting or lying down with the eyes closed or open—gazing softly downward.

How to Practice

In the Zen 10, you count along with your breath:

- Bringing your awareness to the flow of your breath, with the inhalation say to yourself, "Inhale-1." And with the exhalation, say to yourself, "Exhale-1."
- With the next breath, "Inhale-2, exhale-2."
- With the next breath, "Inhale-3, exhale-3." Etc.
- Continue this way of counting all the way up to 10.
- Then with the next breath, start over at one.

It sounds simple, right? Yes and no. As you practice, you may discover that your awareness has wandered to something else, and suddenly you don't know what number you are on. That's okay. When that happens, let go of the thought and return to following the flow of your breath, "Inhale-1."

Or you may discover that you are on a count of 11 or 12. That's okay, too! When that happens, smile to yourself, and go back to, "Inhale-1."

Variation

Some people prefer to have two counts with each cycle of breath. "Inhale-1, exhale-2. Inhale-3, exhale 4," etc. Feel free to count this way if it feels right for you.

Tips

○ In the beginning, because the practice is interesting and new, you may find that it's easy to hold your focus on the numbers and get to 10. But over time, it gets harder. The novelty wears off, and your mind may wander. Don't judge yourself when that happens. Just the opposite. When you notice that you've lost your count, give yourself a high five, smile, and breathe in "one." This discovery that you are lost in other thoughts—and the practice of letting go of those thoughts and coming back to following and counting the breath—strengthens your ability to focus and cultivates present moment awareness. In this way, practicing Zen 10 is like a musician practicing scales. The more you practice, the more facile you get.

○ Some people *love* this practice. It's concrete and clear. Numbers are neutral and don't require any extra thinking. Other people don't connect with this practice at all. They find the numbers to be boring or uninspiring. Both responses are fine, but don't be too quick to judge. Keep an open mind and try the Zen 10 a few times to discover how well it works for you.

1.3. FINGER TRACING

Good for:

- Gathering focus when you are feeling distracted
- Calming the mind
- Coping with anxious thoughts

Introduction

This practice involves physically tracing your hand in time with your breath. It's super simple. As the leader, you'll want to first demonstrate and then invite the group to practice together with you.

How to Practice

- Keeping your eyes open, take one of your hands and spread the fingers out in front of you with your palm up. Place the pointer finger of the other hand at the base of the outside of the thumb.
- Your focus will be on the finger as it traces around your hand.
- As you breathe in, move your pointer finger up the thumb. As you breathe out, trace over and down the inside of the thumb.
- Keep going, tracing your hand all the way to the outside of the pinky finger and then coming all the way back.
- With each inhalation, you'll trace up, and with each exhalation, trace down.
- As you go, breathe deeply and exhale gently. Take your time.

- Try to match the movement with the breath so that you arrive at the top of each finger with the end of each inhalation, and you arrive at the bottom of each finger with the end of each exhalation.

- When you notice your mind is quiet, you may choose to rest your hands in your lap and simply enjoy quiet and easy breathing.

Variation

Notice the pauses in between each inhale and exhale. Pausing for just a fraction of a second at the top of the finger and the base of the finger may help you slow down the breath a little more.

Tips

- Because this exercise is done with eyes open and a focus on the hands, it is especially good for someone who has difficulty "going inside" or for anyone coping with high emotions or anxiety.

- Soothing touch activates our caregiving systems. Just as a hug or pat on the back can soothe and make you feel better, you can generate the same benefits through your own caring touch.

- Here's one practice that doesn't require a timer. Assuming that you slow down your breathing to around five breaths a minute, then you can determine the length of this meditation by choosing the number of rounds you trace your hand. Three times equals six minutes, five times equals 10 minutes, etc.

1.4. BELLY BREATHING

Good for:
- Reducing stress
- Relaxing body and mind

Introduction

When we're stressed, we tend to have shorter and more shallow breathing. You'll get many health benefits from this practice of shifting into deep, slow breathing from the belly—including reduced stress and increased levels of energy.

During Belly Breathing you are consciously controlling the breath. Remember, all controlled breathing should be easy and relaxed. Take your time, and never force the breath.

How to Practice

- Find a comfortable position, either seated or lying down.
- Close the eyes and draw the awareness within.
- Set aside any thoughts as you turn your awareness to the breath.
- Begin by simply observing the breath. Note the quality of the breath—it may be fast or slow, deep or shallow, even or uneven.
- Cultivate a kind and curious awareness of the details of your breath. Don't try to change anything yet. First, notice and accept the breath, just as it is.
- Next, place a hand on the abdomen, and see if you can feel it move with each inhalation and each exhalation—rising and falling. Continue this until you can feel your hand, belly, and breath all connected.

- With the next inhalation, see if you can expand a little more from the belly to take in more air.

- With the next exhalation, see if you can slow down and extend the breath.

- Keeping the breath slow, easy, and gentle, experiment and see how far you can develop this slow, deep breathing.

Variation

Dirgha Swasam, or deep breathing, is a kind of yogic breathing that some people may be familiar with. Also known as the "three-part breath," *Dirgha Swasam* is a natural next step after Belly Breathing. First, you breathe into the abdomen and allow it to expand fully, then continue to inhale expanding the rib cage, and then the upper chest. Then exhale slowly from the upper chest, then the rib cage, and finally the abdomen. The breath should be one continuous, gentle flow.

Tips

- If you are not used to deep breathing, it can feel very challenging at first. Forcing things won't help. Instead, think of relaxing, releasing, or letting go with each exhale. Take your time and focus on breathing in a way that's gentle and easy.

- To slow down the breath, when you think you are at the end of your exhale, see if maybe you can exhale just a little bit more. It might help to think of drawing the navel toward the spine.

1.5. SLOWING DOWN THE EXHALE (AKA 4:2:6)

Good for:

- Relaxing body and mind
- Health benefits such as reducing blood pressure

Introduction

The 4:2:6 breath involves breathing in for a count of four, holding the breath for a count of two, and exhaling for a count of six. The key to this practice is slowing down the exhale so that it is longer than the inhale. Why? Because the respiratory system and the nervous system are closely connected. When we relax the body, our breath automatically slows down. The opposite is also true. When we consciously slow down the exhale, the body relaxes. Specifically, the parasympathetic nervous system engages—slowing down the heart rate and releasing hormones that send the body into a state of "rest and digest."

The 4:2:6 breath creates the conditions for your body to repair and heal.

How to Practice

- Find a comfortable position, either seated or lying down.

- Close the eyes and draw the awareness within.

- Set aside any thoughts as you turn your awareness to the breath.

- Cultivate a kind and curious awareness of the details of your breath. Don't try to change anything yet. First, notice and accept the breath just as it is.

- Next, start to count your inhalation at whatever pace is comfortable for you. For example, you may find that your inhale lasts for two or three counts.

- Relax your breathing until your inhale lasts for four counts, "Inhale-2-3-4."

- Once you have a count established, start to match the length of your exhalation with the same count as your inhalation. For example, "Inhale-2-3-4 and exhale-2-3-4."

- Once you settle into this rhythm, you may find that it's possible to slow down the exhale. Take your time and work toward a *comfortable* rhythm, inhaling for four and exhaling for six.

- *If it's comfortable*, you can then add a pause. At the top of the inhale, hold for two counts. For example, "Inhale-2-3-4, pause-2, exhale-2-3-4-5-6."

- Try this exercise for about five or 10 minutes. When your mind wanders, don't worry. Just notice that it has happened and return your focus to counting and easy breathing.

Variation

There are many different techniques for controlling the breath that have been popularized, including the 4:7:8 breath and "box breathing," which involve holding in and holding out the breath for longer periods of time. I do *not* recommend these techniques unless you have a regular breathing practice and can do these comfortably. You should never force or strain, feel dizzy or light-headed, or be gasping for air during a breath practice.

Tips

- The reason to hold the breath is to create focus and further relaxation. It might help to think "relax," instead of "pause," as you count. For example, "Inhale-2-3-4, *relax*-2, exhale-2-3-4-5-6." The goal is to experience a moment of stillness and peace, so if holding your breath feels uncomfortable, don't do it!

- If all the counting feels too busy, drop the count and simply focus on slowing down the exhale. Think of relaxing, releasing, or letting go with each exhale until you have a general sense that your exhalation is longer than your inhalation.

1.6. COHERENT BREATHING

Good for:
- Calming the body
- Promoting relaxation and healing

Introduction

Coherent breathing is a breath-based practice where you consciously control the breath to make your inhalations and exhalations equal in length.

You can practice this meditation sitting or lying down with the eyes closed.

How to Practice

Begin by closing the eyes and drawing your awareness within. Set aside worries, plans, and other thoughts.

- Bring your attention to the sensations of breathing. Perhaps you'll notice the air flowing in and out of the nostrils, or your chest or belly rising and falling.

- Cultivate a kind and curious awareness of the details of your breath. Don't try to change anything yet. First, notice and accept the breath just as it is.

- Next, start to count your inhalation at whatever pace is comfortable for you. For example, you may find that your inhale lasts for two or three counts.

- Once you have a count established, start to match the length of your exhalation with the same count as your inhalation. For example, "Inhale-2-3 and exhale-2-3." Take your time to find a rhythm that is *comfortable* for you.

- As you settle into this rhythm, you may find that it's possible to slow down the breath and relax a little more. *If it's comfortable*, you can either slow down the speed of your count, or you can add more numbers to your count (for example, "Inhale-2-3-4 and exhale-2-3-4").

- Try this exercise for about five or 10 minutes. When your mind wanders, don't worry. Just notice that it has happened and return to paying attention to your breath and making it even and consistent.

Variation

Paying attention to your breath is a great exercise because it's something you can do anytime and anywhere—standing in line, lying in bed, sitting at your desk, or even driving your car.

Tips

- Making a conscious effort to equalize your breathing takes focus. When you pay close attention to the details of your breath, create a rhythmic flow, and slow down, the thoughts will also slow down.

- The breath is connected to the nervous system. Slowing down the breath switches on your parasympathetic nervous system (sometimes referred to as the system of "rest-and-digest"). This also slows the heart rate and relaxes the body.

- Most people take about 10 to 14 breaths each minute. Slowing down the breath to about six breaths over the course of a minute (that's equal to five seconds for each inhale and five seconds for each exhale) is the point at which the parasympathetic nervous system turns on.

○ The purpose of this practice is to relax and relieve stress. If you notice you are forcing the breath or feel uncomfortable, then let go. Stop trying to control things and return to feeling the sensations of breathing and accepting the breath just as it is. Let your breathing be easy. Sometimes the breath is short or shallow, and that's okay.

"Breathe in deeply
to bring your mind
home to your body"

THICH NHAT HANH

1.7. WATCHING THE CYCLES OF BREATHING

Good for:

- Developing focus and a clear mind
- Cultivating a non-judgmental state of mind
- Finding peace and joy

Introduction

In this practice, you place your awareness on the flow of the breath in the present moment—watching the breath with focus and care. In time, you may arrive at a state of being that is both relaxed and alert that brings pleasure, ease, and peace.

How to Practice

- Sitting comfortably, draw the awareness within. Relax the face and shoulders.

- Shift your awareness from the body and begin to observe the breath.

- Notice the details of the breath—fast, slow, shallow, deep, even, uneven, etc.

- Notice the physical sensations of breathing in the body. Do you feel the belly going in and out, the rib cage expanding and relaxing, the air as it passes through the nostrils or the throat?

- Set aside other thoughts and give your complete attention to the breath. (*Pause for a minute or two.*)

- Now, begin to observe the cycle of breathing.

    - Notice the inhalation.

    - Then a pause, a moment of transition.

- Follow the breath through the exhalation.
- Then a brief moment of emptiness.
- And the birth of the new breath, an impulse to inhale.

- Take on a curious attitude and see what details you can discover about your breath.

- No two breaths are the same. See if you can stay present and notice the complete cycle of the breath. Pay special attention to the transitions. Can you notice the exact moment when the inhale begins? And the slight pause between inhale and exhale?

- When you notice that your thoughts have shifted to something else, that's an important and powerful moment. Celebrate that you noticed it, let go of the thought, and return your attention back to the breath.

Variation

For some people, it helps their focus to put their attention on something very specific, such as the feeling of the air flowing in and out of the nostrils. For others, imagery helps them keep their focus. For example, you might imagine your breath as gentle waves washing in and out of the shore. It's fine to adapt and take an approach that feels comfortable for you.

Tips

- Be patient with yourself as you learn how to isolate your attention on the present moment through the breath. Mindfulness will come and go. Your first assignment is to know when it's present and when it's gone. Be watchful and discover how your mind moves. Then, learn how to reestablish mindfulness—adjust your posture, pay attention to the sensory events of the breath, or smile to yourself.

o You may notice thoughts like, "*This is boring. This is hard. I can't do this.*" Observe those stories, but don't get involved with them. Simply keep practicing, dropping thoughts, and focusing on the breath.

Source: This practice is adapted from the teachings of Rich Panico, MD.

HOW TO REESTABLISH MINDFULNESS WHEN YOU LOSE IT

It's easy to say, "Let go of thoughts," but not so easy to do. The practice is not to be continuously mindful. That's very, very difficult. It takes a long time for that to happen. The practice is mindfulness coming and going and working with that coming and going. When members of your group report that their mind is busy, or they are having trouble focusing, here are a few suggestions you can offer that might help.

① Be kind

When a baby is learning how to walk, do you get mad at them when they fall down? Of course not! Falling down is part of the learning process. When you feel frustrated, try applying the kind of loving encouragement that you would give to a little child. Smile, and try giving yourself some encouragement like, "Oh look, I'm thinking about _____. My brain is so interesting. Now I'm going to pick up the practice again."

② Check your posture

Whenever the mind wanders, and especially when you feel sleepy, you can always bring awareness to the posture. Are you slumping? Is there tension or tightness somewhere that you can relax? Adjusting the posture can help reset or refocus the mind.

A common instruction you may hear is to "sit in a way that's dignified, like a mountain." Any image or quality that signals the brain to be alert, without clenching or forcing, is a good one. I have a teacher that uses the image of a "300-pound linebacker holding a sleeping baby" to describe the combination of power and gentleness necessary to be in present-moment awareness.

③ Connect to an anchor

Refer to Chapter 3 on the usefulness of a personal anchor as a way to reestablish mindfulness.

④ Let go of judgments

Be on watch for judgments—thoughts like right or wrong, good or bad, should or can't. We all have judgments. During practice note them, watch them, but don't get involved with them. Imagine you are watching a movie and there is a critic sitting next to you judging each scene. Give your attention to the movie, not the critic.

It doesn't matter if the mind is being super active. Just note, without judgment, that the mind is being active, and watch it.

(5) Remember, it's a practice

If you want to get good at basketball, you have to practice shooting the ball—not just once or twice but over and over. If you want to experience more presence and peace, you have to practice it repeatedly.

Loss of mindfulness occurs. In fact, it's anticipated and welcomed wholeheartedly. These interruptions of mindfulness and reasserting of mindfulness give you the opportunity to strengthen your skills. Give it time and you will see results.

Section 2:
Body-Based Practices

Just like the breath, the body is a key pathway to achieving calm, focus, and peace. In fact, the mind, body, and breath are connected. If you slow down the breath, the body will automatically relax. And if you relax the body, the breath will automatically slow down. Both actions support a slowing down of thoughts and a relaxing of the mind, which can lead to greater focus, calm, and presence.

These practices are good for beginners, because the body is tangible, and it's always with us. Focusing on the body gets us out of our heads.

In addition, our bodies are a source of valuable information that we often ignore. Paying attention to your body can be an important way to be more responsive to your physical and emotional health. Body-based practices are therefore extremely useful to help ease stress, support healing, and improve mood.

2.1. BODY SCAN

Good for:

- Reducing stress
- Relaxing body and mind
- Opening to the present moment

Introduction

We often go through our days without paying careful and caring attention to our bodies, which are fundamental to our existence. This practice is an act of self-care. It involves systematically moving attention through the body, connecting with the direct experience of sensation from the inside out.

How to Practice

Sitting or lying in a comfortable position, begin by taking two or three deep breaths—inhaling through the nose and exhaling through the mouth. Then, allow your breathing to settle into its own rhythm, breathing in *and out* through the nose.

For the next few minutes, set aside your thoughts and give all your attention to your physical body. There are two guidelines:

1. **Be curious.** Explore sensations in different parts of your body. There's no right or wrong; just observe and discover whatever you can.

2. **Be kind.** Bring an intention to really care for your body during this practice.

- To start, bring your awareness to your left foot and notice any sensations—such as the pressure on the sole of the foot if it's resting on the floor or the feeling of a sock touching the skin.

- Next, focus on the left leg from the ankle all the way up to the hip. What sensations do you notice?

- Bring awareness to the right foot and right leg. Be curious and see what sensations you can discover. Are the sensations similar or different from your left foot and leg?

- Move your awareness to your left hand, arm, and shoulder....Do you notice any feeling of heaviness or tension? If you can, perhaps bring relaxation to the left arm.

- Next, be aware of sensations in your right hand, arm, and shoulder....Perhaps relaxing them a little bit.

- Use your awareness to scan the lower back, middle back, upper back, and shoulder blades. Feel the natural curves of the back and any sensations in the back.

- Then scan your belly, rib cage, and upper chest. Can you feel the sensations of breathing? Notice the quality of your breath and, maybe, slow down the breath.

- Bring your awareness to your neck and jaw. Notice any tension and perhaps relax the jaw, the mouth and tongue. And then the cheeks, the muscles around the eyes and behind the eyes.

- Be aware of any sensations in your forehead, the top of your head and back of the head.

- Finally, expand your awareness to include the whole body. If you notice any tension, explore and see if you can bring relaxation.

- To end, take a few deeper breaths. Then come back to an awareness of the space around you, and when you're ready, open your eyes.

Variations

There are many ways to lead a body scan. In this practice, awareness moves from the feet to the head. It's also fine to start with the head and end with the feet.

A body scan can be limited to just observing sensation, or it can include an invitation to bring relaxation and/or healing to different parts of the body. Explore and find the right approach that works for you and your group.

Tips

o Take time to allow people to tune into sensations. Be sure to pause and give at least five to 10 seconds on each area of the body before moving to the next.

o Remember, everyone's experience is different and okay. Words like "perhaps" or "maybe" invite possibility and avoid forcing any particular experience.

o Thich Nhat Hanh used the phrase "I smile to my body" as a way to invoke loving-kindness toward oneself.

o Maintaining focus on the physical body can be challenging and triggering for people who are coping with—or have a history of—injury, physical pain, disease, abuse, and/or trauma. Remind people they can always drop the body scan and return to an anchor if they feel discomfort or difficult emotion.

o Learning to relax the body is a useful skill to develop that will get easier with practice.

o Complement this practice with the poem "Do Not Go to the Garden of Flowers" by Kabir.

2.2. WORKING WITH PHYSICAL PAIN

Good for:

o Learning to manage and cope with physical pain

Introduction

If you are working with a group in a healthcare or medical setting, you may have people ask what to do when they have acute or chronic pain. Here's a practice that you can offer to those who are looking for ways to cope with pain.

Often, we try to wall off pain, or resist it, or try not to think about it. In this practice, you go in the other direction and take a detailed look at the nature of your pain. This practice is not for the faint of heart. As a leader, show compassion for each person's experience and acknowledge that it takes courage to open up to physical pain.

How to Practice

Sitting or lying in a comfortable position, begin by taking two or three deep breaths—inhaling through the nose and exhaling through the mouth. Then allow your breathing to settle into its own rhythm, breathing in *and out* through the nose.

o Start by labeling the breath—silently saying to yourself, "Inhale/exhale," or, "In/out," as you breathe. Use your breath as an anchor. Anytime you get distracted or simply need to take a break, you can come back here and focus on the breath.

o Scan the entire body and notice where you feel the pain. Pick one area of the body and observe the sensations you feel there.

- Imagine that you are a reporter and it's your job to give as much detail as possible about what's happening. Is the pain sharp or throbbing? Does it feel hot or tight? Does it stay in one place, or does it move around? Does the intensity change over time?

- Next, create an image that represents this pain. It might be a cloud of electricity that sends out angry sparks, or it might be a hard, black rock, or a heavy weight. Settle on one image for right now.

- How could your image of the pain be transformed? Can you imagine rain falling and the storm passing? Or the rock dissolving into sand? Or putting the weight into an aquamarine pool of tropical water where it can float?

- There's no right or wrong image. Go with whatever occurs to you—it doesn't matter if it's silly or nonsensical. Notice what you can change about the image of your pain. The color? The material? The temperature?

- When you're ready, bring your awareness back to the breath.

- Scan through the body and see if you notice any changes.

- Whether you experience some change or no change at all, appreciate your effort and the courage that it takes to face the pain.

- Take a deep breath in. Let it out. And then open your eyes.

Variation

Some people have vivid imaginations; they can easily create images in their minds. For others, it can be more difficult—and for a small percentage it's impossible because their brains are not wired to create mental pictures. If you can't come up with an image, simply continue observing the sensations in the body.

Tips

- Observing pain doesn't make it go away. Yet, taking the perspective of an outside reporter, or observer, of your own pain creates a bit of separation. When there's an awareness separate from the pain, you've created a part of you that's not identified with the pain. To help people create this kind of separation, you might try adding some questions like, "Who holds the pain? What happens when no one holds the pain?"

- Sometimes chronic pain can feel constant, but as the saying goes: "The only constant in life is change." Noticing even slight fluctuations in the pain's severity can bring a little relief.

- Complement this practice with the poems "Let This Darkness Be a Bell Tower" by Rainer Maria Rilke or "Paradox of Noise" by Gunilla Norris.

Source: This practice is adapted from *Detox Your Thoughts* by Andrea Bonior, PhD.

"Research has shown that mindfulness interventions increase pain tolerance. By fully facing and acknowledging our experience, we make it less frightening and intense, even though we assume that the opposite would be true."

ANDREA BONIOR, PHD

2.3. WALKING MEDITATION

Good for:

o   Anyone who has difficulty sitting still
o   Coping with anxious thoughts

Introduction

Walking meditation is a very ancient practice that goes all the way back to the time of the Buddha. In walking meditation, you step in time with your breath. With each inhale, raise the heel of your back foot. Exhale as you plant your foot forward in front of you.

To do walking meditation with a group, you'll need to have enough room to move around—usually walking as a group in a circle. Explain and demonstrate this for the group first, and then have everyone join in.

How to Practice

o   Stand up. Keep your eyes open and look downward with a soft focus on what's ahead of you. Feel your feet in contact with the ground.

o   Decide how you want to hold your hands. You can have them at your sides. You can interlace your fingers in front of you. You can have your hands behind you and hold onto your wrist with the opposite hand. Find a comfortable position for your arms and hands so you don't have to think about them.

o   Inhale and raise one heel up. Keep your toes on the floor—it's not a balancing act. As you exhale, you move the foot forward and transfer your weight. Then, inhale and pick up your other heel. As you exhale, move the foot forward. That's the whole thing. You are inhaling and exhaling with each step.

o The pace will vary depending on the length of your breath, and that's okay. Generally, you'll be going slowly.

o Walk in a circle and follow the leader. You're all the leader, and you're all the followers. You're all equal. If you notice you are taking bigger steps than the person in front of you, take smaller steps. You don't need to get anywhere. You can do this by walking in place.

o To finish, find a chair, sit, and close your eyes. See if you can keep your breathing going at the same rhythm, sitting.

o And finally, you can open your eyes.

Variations

Walking meditation can be done indoors or outdoors. If there's not enough room to walk in a circle, you can walk back and forth in a line. You only need 10–20 feet of space. You can even step in place.

For someone who is unable to walk, you can "walk" with your hands. Sit and put your hands on your thighs. Pick up one hand and put it back down in time with the breath. Establish a rhythm of breathing and move the hands just as you would move the feet if you were walking.

If you want, you can repeat a mantra or an affirmation along with each step. For example, inhale and say to yourself, "Deep," and exhale saying, "Slow." Or try, "Be here (inhale) now (exhale)."

Tips

○ Anything with a rhythm can help you with your meditation. You can get into a meditative rhythm while walking, jogging, or swimming.

○ The goal isn't to get somewhere. The goal is to get to a quiet mind, using the rhythm to help you.

○ You can use this technique throughout the day. Anytime you are walking—if you have something important to think about, think about that. But if you have "*blah blah blah*" going on in your head, use that time to practice. Of course, in daily life you want to walk faster than you do during walking meditation, so you'll need to adjust your pace. Instead of taking a single breath with each step, try taking three or four steps with each inhalation and exhalation.

2.4. INSIDE OUTSIDE

Good for:
- Quieting a busy mind
- Reducing stress

Introduction

In this playful practice, we move our awareness using the sensations in different areas of the body as a focus. It invites us to experience the body and use our brain in new ways— ways that shift us from thinking to feeling. This type of body sensing activates a natural relaxation response throughout your body.

How to Practice

- Sit in a comfortable position and close the eyes.

- Breathe slowly through your nose and begin sensing your body, knowing that whatever you experience is perfect just as it is.

- Feel the places where your body is in contact with the floor or chair. Feel any sensations in the bottoms of your feet. Notice the pressure in your seat as gravity roots you to the ground, pulling you toward the earth.

- Adjust your posture. Allow your spine to elongate and feel the top of the head rising toward the sky.

- Notice both feelings together—drawing down toward the ground and rising up toward the sky. *Allow some extra time in silence here.*

- Next, move your attention to the left side of your body. Notice any sensations you feel in your left leg, arm, or hand. This could be feelings of temperature or tingling. Be curious and see what you can feel.

o Let go of the left side and bring awareness to the sensations on the right side of your body. Scan the right side of your body and see what sensations you notice.

o Then, take a few breaths with an awareness of both sides of the body. *Allow some extra time in silence here.*

o Move the attention to the front of your body. What sensations and movement do you feel in the belly, rib cage, collar bones? Feel the movement and sensation on the front side of your body.

o Then shift to an awareness of your back. Scan the lower back, middle back, and upper back. Does your back also move with the breath? What other sensations do you feel?

o Expand your awareness now to include both the front and back of the body. Feel the torso as a whole— expanding and relaxing with the breath. *Allow some extra time in silence here.*

o Finally, see if you can sense the space inside your body.

o Then, shift focus and see if you can sense the space around you, outside of your body.

o Merge and feel your awareness of the space both inside and outside the body.

o Feel yourself as open and aware. Sense any feeling of security, peace, and well-being. *Allow some extra time in silence here.*

o Notice and appreciate any relaxation you've experienced during this practice.

o When you are ready, gently open your eyes and return to the room.

Variation

This practice explores shifting awareness down/up, left/right, front/back, and inside/outside. If you only have a few minutes, you can shorten this to just a couple directions. For example, down/up followed by inside/outside. Or left/right and front/back.

Tips

- In this exercise, it may feel silly to suggest that someone can feel the space outside of themselves. Is that even possible? You won't know until you try! This kind of novel instruction causes our brains to fire in new ways.

- Giving instructions that are unexpected can stretch our normal way of thinking. For example, during deep relaxation my yoga teacher will often give instructions to relax the nose. I'm pretty sure the nose is made of cartilage and that there are no muscles there to relax. But the act of *trying* brings a quality of concentration and curiosity.

Source: This practice is inspired by the work of iRest founder, Dr. Robert Miller.

2.5. CLOUD HANDS

Good for:

- Beginners
- Gathering focus when you are feeling distracted
- Calming the body and mind

Introduction

Cloud Hands is a practice that combines a focus on the body along with the breath. It's inspired by Qigong, an ancient Chinese practice that uses mindful movements and breathing to connect mind, body, and spirit.

This practice involves moving the hands up and down with the breath like they are moving through clouds. As the leader, demonstrate the movement and then invite the group to practice together with you.

How to Practice

- Either seated or standing, and with your eyes open, make sure your feet are flat on the floor about shoulder width apart.
- Hold your hands with the palms facing up. If you are seated, the backs of your hands will be resting on your lap. If you are standing, have your elbows bent with the hands waist high.
- As you breath, you'll move your hands up and down— slowing and smoothly, as if you are moving through clouds.
- Inhale bringing the hands up to shoulder height.
- As you transition to exhale, turn the palms downward and allow the hands to float back down.

- As the exhale ends, turn the palms upward and raise the hands in time with your next inhalation.
- Continue moving the hands in this way, in conjunction with the breath.
- Go at your own pace.
- Try to match the movement with the breath so that you arrive at the top just as you finish each inhalation, and you arrive at the bottom at the end of each exhalation.
- At any time, you may choose to rest your hands in your lap or at your sides and simply enjoy quiet and easy breathing.

Variation

Once your group is comfortable with this basic movement, you can change the hand movements so that they alternate—with the right hand going up as the left hand comes down and the left hand coming up as the right hand goes down. At first, it may feel like trying to pat your head and rub your belly at the same time. It'll take a little practice for this movement to flow naturally, which is a good thing. The extra challenge will help focus the mind.

Tips

- This seems like a simple practice, but coordinating the movement of your hands in time with the breath takes real concentration. To make the movement smooth and steady requires attention and control, leaving no room to think about anything else.
- Because this exercise is done with eyes open and a focus on the hands, it is especially good for someone who has difficulty "going inside" or for anyone coping with high emotions or anxiety.

2.6. GROUNDING LIKE A TREE

Good for:
- o Centering attention
- o Increasing connection

Introduction

This practice involves a focus on the body combined with visualizations of the natural world. Images from nature are used to cultivate qualities of steadiness, strength, and vitality. This is adapted from the work of my friend and nature connection guide, Kai Siedenburg, who uses nature awareness as a path to mind-body wellness.

How to Practice

- o Find a comfortable position, allowing your eyes to close or lowering your gaze.

- o Bring your awareness inside, noticing that you are in a body and your body is breathing—two amazing things that we sometimes take for granted.

- o Rest your awareness on the breath, allowing that to invite you into the present moment, into your own body.

- o Scan through the body. If anything feels tight or uncomfortable, see if you can allow it to soften or release.

- o If your body wants to stretch or move a little, I invite you to do that.

- o *Pause.*

- Now bring your awareness to your feet, maybe pressing them into the floor or wiggling your toes. Feeling your feet.

- Sense the presence of the living Earth beneath your feet—including the ground, soil, rock, and water beneath the building that you are in. Opening your awareness to the earth.

- If it feels right for you, you can sense energetic roots extending from your feet down into the earth—as far as you want. Let the roots travel down into the earth.

- Open yourself to receive energy and nourishment from the Earth in this moment, allowing that energy to flow into you and nourish you.

- Now, gently shift awareness to the top of your head, the crown. Then, open your awareness to the sky above— the vast spaciousness of the sky, the stars, and galaxies.

- Feel yourself here, rooted in the earth, open to the sky and heavens, balanced like a tree.

- You might imagine your favorite tree and become that tree—strong, grounded, steady, and vibrant.

- As we get ready to transition back to this circle, notice your breath and your body again. Maybe moving and stretching.

- As you are ready, gently allow your eyes to open.

Variation

Connecting with nature, even if only in our minds, can be a path to greater peace, joy, and balance. It can also open us to gratitude. If appropriate for your group, you can invite a moment of gratitude before ending the practice:

- Notice something or someone that you feel grateful for in this moment. It could be anything. Just notice what comes—feeling it and sending some gratitude and appreciation. Saying "thank you" if that feels right.

Tips

- Visualizations come more naturally for some people than for others. Encourage the members of your group to keep their visualization simple. It's okay to focus on broad ideas rather than trying to "see" every leaf of their tree.

- Complement this practice with the poem "When I Am Among the Trees" by Mary Oliver. Or, share this quote with your group:

> "Even a wounded world is feeding us.
> Even a wounded world holds us, giving us
> moments of wonder and joy. I choose joy over
> despair. Not because I have my head in the
> sand, but because joy is what the earth gives
> me daily and I must return the gift."

ROBIN WALL KIMMERER, *BRAIDING SWEETGRASS*

———————

Source: Kai Siedenburg, nature connection guide, ecotherapist, and author of the series *Poems of Earth and Spirit*.

VISUALIZATION

Visualization is a powerful tool that has been well studied as a method to improve performance or to enhance healing. Focusing on an image during a meditation or mindfulness practice helps move us out of discursive thinking to an awareness beyond words. Visualization also activates neural pathways that can change our physical state.

In the case of the Grounding Like a Tree practice above, drawing on images of the earth, sky, and trees can help people cultivate embodied qualities, like stability and courage, that are hard to arrive at through the intellect.

Visualization is also key to many of the compassion practices included in section 5.0 of this chapter. Research on Loving-Kindness Meditation, which involves thinking of a person connected with loving-kindness, has revealed measurable changes in the brain, specifically in areas responsible for empathy and emotional intelligence.[23]

Section 3:
Focused Awareness Practices

In focused awareness practices, just as the name suggests, you pick something specific to focus on—sometimes called an "object of concentration." The practices described in the previous two sections invite concentration on the breath and body. The practices in this section include other possible points of focus.

Why might you want to focus awareness? It's all about quieting the mind and reaching a state that is calm and peaceful—beyond thought. Creating thoughts is a natural thing that the mind does—and so the mind wanders. It might be scanning the environment to notice what's happening around you, or it might be contemplating events in the past, planning for the future, or imagining something outside of reality altogether.

Having thoughts is not a problem. But having out-of-control thoughts, or becoming too identified with our thoughts, can be problematic. With focused awareness practices we learn how to work with the thoughts. One of the best ways to separate from our thoughts is to pick one thing to focus on. I like to think of the mind like the trunk of an elephant. The elephant's trunk wanders and explores its environment all the time, but if you give the elephant a stick to hold in its trunk, it will stop wandering.

Our minds are similar. When we give the mind something specific to hold onto, we steady thinking on one thing, and the other thoughts drop away. Of course, this won't happen immediately. During focused awareness practices, the mind will wander off. Learning to steady the mind means noticing and returning awareness to the object of concentration over and over again. Explore the practices in this section with your group to see how this works.

3.1. USING A MANTRA

Good for:

o Steadying the mind

Introduction

A mantra is a word or phrase that you repeat over and over as an object of focused concentration. Did you ever read the children's book *The Little Engine That Could*? If you did, you probably remember the refrain of that book: "I think I can. I think I can. I think I can." This is a great example of a mantra.

The word mantra literally means a "tool of thought" (from Sanskrit "manas" (mind) and "tra" (tool). In ancient traditions going back more than 3,000 years, especially in the yoga traditions, there are specific mantras that hold divine vibration, such as "OM" or "Rama." (Rama was Gandhi's mantra.)

But any words can work. Keep it simple, uplifting, and/or meaningful. A mantra isn't a prayer or a hope. It clarifies or concentrates an intent. Pick something that you like. Some examples include:

o Thank you

o Here now

o Coming home

o Relaxed, at peace

o Peace, joy, love, and light

o Present moment, beautiful moment

How to Practice

A mantra is typically repeated silently in rhythm with the breath.

- Begin in a seated position and close your eyes.

- Adjust your posture so you are comfortable, and then move your attention to your breath. Observe the natural rhythm of your inhale and exhale.

- Then, begin repeating your mantra in time with the breath. Find a flow that works for you. This might mean that the mantra is divided between the inhale and exhale, or that you repeat it completely with each inhale and again with each exhale.

- Sometimes the mind will wander. You'll notice you are thinking about something else and have dropped the mantra. When you notice that, let go of the thought and begin repeating the mantra again.

Variations

In addition to silently repeating a mantra in your head, you can silently mouth the words or speak it aloud if that helps you maintain your focus. You can also use pen and paper and write the mantra over and over.

Tip

- Repeating a mantra is something you can do throughout the day—when you are washing dishes, taking a shower, or going for a walk.

3.2. GAZING

Good for:

- Moving beyond thought
- Anyone who is uncomfortable "going inside"

Introduction

Gazing practice, also known as *Tratak*, involves using an image as an object of concentration. This might be the flame of a candle, or a flower, a mandala, or any image or object that is meaningful. Just like a mantra, whatever object you choose should be simple, uplifting, and meaningful.

How to Practice

- Place your image or object at eye height.
- Then, close the eyes and take a few deep breaths—in through the nose and out through the mouth.
- Allow the breath to settle into its own natural rhythm, and then open the eyes.
- Look at your object with a soft gaze. The eyes should be relaxed.
- Notice the whole of the object.
- Next, explore the individual details of the object.
- When you feel that you can remember what it looks like, close your eyes and imagine the object with your eyes closed.
- When your mind wanders, you can open your eyes, and there it is. Look at your object. Get inspiration from it. Remember it and close your eyes. Once again, hold the image in your mind's eye.

- If the object has a meaning for you, focus on the idea behind the object.
- To bring the practice to a close, take a few deeper breaths.
- Notice any effects this practice has had on the state of your body and mind.

Variation

When you close your eyes, you can experiment with the location of your visualization. You might continue to see the image in front of you, or you can imagine the image within yourself. For example, if you are gazing at a candle, you might imagine warmth and light radiating inside your body. If you are gazing at a flower or an object from nature, you might imagine your connection with nature and all of life. See if you can feel the qualities of your image inside your body.

Tips

- Keep the object at eye level or slightly above. You want to be in a posture that helps you stay alert and awake— not looking down.
- With gazing, you let go of thinking and focus on a visual image instead. Experiment and see if you can become absorbed with the senses and your direct experience without needing any words.
- Bring candles or other objects for people to use during this practice. Or if you have a regular group, invite people to bring an object or image that's meaningful to them.

3.3. COUNTING BACKWARD

Good for:
- Quieting a busy mind
- Focus/concentration

Introduction

You'll find my favorite counting meditation, the Zen 10, as Practice 1.2 under Breath-Based Practices. (Most counting practices are also breath practices—unless you are in bed counting sheep.)

This practice isn't as simple as the Zen 10, but the extra complexity can be a good thing—keeping the mind focused.

How to Practice

- You'll be counting down from 30. With your next inhale, start at 30.

- Then exhale 29. Inhale 28 and exhale 27, etc.

- When you get to 10, slow down the count so there's a full round of breath for each number. So you'll inhale 10 and exhale 10. Then inhale nine, exhale nine, etc.

- When you get to one, notice if your mind is quiet. If it is, just rest and breathe and appreciate this peace. If it's not, that's okay. Return to 30 and repeat the countdown.

- There will be times you get carried away by other thoughts and lose your count. When this happens, you can either return to the last number you remember and start there, or you can start at 30 again.

Variation

There are many variations of counting as a way to focus the mind. Another is to simply count backward from 100 to 0, or backwards by multiples of 5 or 3, or other intervals.

Feel free to invent your own.

Tip

- Some people's first reaction to counting is that numbers are "cold" or "rational," and they believe that counting can't be relaxing. Give it a try anyway. You may be surprised at how effective counting can be. It's direct and simple. There's no need for extra thinking, and our brains like that.

Source: I learned this practice from a fellow meditation teacher, Kelley Annese, who adapted it from the work of Erich Schiffmann.[24]

Section 4:
Open Awareness Practices

Open awareness practices rely on the concept of mindfulness, which was popularized in the West during the 1970s, alongside growing interest in Eastern philosophies. Cultivating open awareness involves bringing attention to present-moment experience with kindness and without judgment. In focused awareness, as described in the previous section, you direct attention to something specific. In open awareness, you focus on whatever is happening in the moment—what's happening *now* is your focus. This is sometimes referred to as "witness consciousness."

A brilliant analogy to describe the difference between focused and open awareness is found in the book *Search Inside Yourself* by Chade-Meng Tan. He likens focused awareness to a closely guarded royal palace where only the most-honored guests are allowed to enter, and all others are courteously but firmly turned away. By contrast, open awareness is like an open house with a friendly host, where anyone who walks in is welcomed as an honored guest.

The practices in this section will help you be connected and in tune with yourself and your surroundings as a witness, without adding assumptions or judgments. Decades of scientific study on the effects of mindfulness practices show resounding evidence that these practices benefit health and well-being, resulting in:

- Increased empathy/compassion
- Decreased anxiety and stress
- Improved sleep and reduced fatigue
- Reduced ruminating thoughts
- Improved tolerance of physical pain
- Lessened depression
- Improved immune functioning
- Improved resilience[25]

Open awareness requires kindness, curiosity, and compassion. It's also effective in fostering creativity and new insight.

4.1. AWARENESS OF YOUR ENVIRONMENT

Good for:

- Beginners
- Cultivating a curious and nonjudgemental state of mind
- Breaking away from anxiety or intense emotions

Introduction

There are many methods you can use to connect to the present moment with open awareness. The five senses of sight, hearing, touch, taste, and smell offer a range of possibilities. Below are a couple different examples you can try.

Slowing down to pay attention to your environment calms your brain. This, in turn, prepares you to engage with the world more effectively and compassionately.

How to Practice

① Colors Around You

Pick a color, maybe orange. Then look around your environment and notice and name all things that are orange. "A *book cover, the cord attached to my computer, etc.*" Then pick another color, maybe green. And again, name all the things around you of that color. "*The leaves of the African violet, the grass in the photo hanging on my wall, the label on the water bottle, etc.*" Be thorough and deliberate as you focus on different colors.

② Sounds Around You

Close your eyes and pay attention to the sounds around you. From moment to moment, notice and name the different sounds that may come and go. For example, *"I hear a car going by on the street outside, the hum of my computer, my roommate typing on the other side of the wall, my stomach gurgling. There goes another car, etc."*

Variation

Rather than focusing on a single sense, such as sight or hearing, you can guide a group to pay attention to each of the five senses sequentially.

Tips

- If you are holding a meeting outdoors or in a beautiful location, this is an especially good practice to use.

- Complement this practice with the poem "Lost" by David Wagoner.

- Suggest to your group that they can use these exercises any time they want to feel more present. For example, before beginning a task, they can stop, close their eyes, and listen to the sounds around them to help them clear their mind. Or when sitting in a waiting room, they can scan for objects of different colors to help them stay calm.

4.2. OBSERVING THOUGHTS

Good for:

- Increasing self-awareness
- Developing self-compassion

Introduction

With practice, we can learn to loosen the hold of thoughts and create space and perspective—giving our minds a rest from the busy stream of thoughts. An important first step is cultivating an open awareness of what's happening inside. This practice provides an opportunity to befriend our thoughts, instead of pushing the thoughts away.

Before you begin, remind your group that having thoughts is normal and okay! Ask them to set an intention to cultivate a friendly attitude toward their minds—observing thoughts with kindness and curiosity (not frustration or judgment).

How to Practice

- Start by drawing your awareness within. Close your eyes or lower your gaze.
- Bring your awareness to how you are sitting.
- Scan the body. Notice any tension and adjust the body to get comfortable.
- Notice the breath and any sensations of breathing. There's nothing to do. Nothing to change. Just witness the breath as it is.
- As you sit and breathe, you will notice different thoughts coming up. Be a witness to the thoughts. Be curious and see what appears.

- Don't fight the thoughts, but don't follow them either. Once you notice the thought, summarize it by describing the thought to yourself. For example, "I'm thinking about what happened yesterday." Or "I'm thinking about my dog." Or "I'm thinking about how many things I need to get done today."

- Then, let go of the thought and return to simply breathing... until you notice another thought. When the next thought comes, describe that thought and allow it to pass like a cloud passing through the vast blue sky.

- Let the thoughts come. Let them go. Watch, but don't get attached. Use the breath as an anchor—coming back to the breath when you get caught up in thoughts.

- Be both kind and curious as you observe the different thoughts. Notice if they are coming rapidly or slowly. Are they mostly thoughts of the past or the future? Do they jump around, or are they fixed on something?

- There's no right or wrong, no good or bad. "Right and wrong, good and bad" are just more thoughts. Notice them, and then let them go.

- End with a moment of gratitude—appreciating your brain, and all its thoughts, as well as your body, and your whole self.

Variations

When watching your thoughts, you can develop a shorthand for labeling them. For example, the labels "past" and "future" will cover 90% of most people's thoughts. Or you might use labels, such as thinking, planning, remembering, worrying, dreaming, etc. However you choose to label the thoughts, choose something that is simple and doesn't require too much effort.

You can add various visualizations to this practice. For example, you might imagine that you are taking off in an airplane on a cloudy, gray day. Eventually you rise above the clouds and see the sun shining in a blue sky. Take this 30,000-foot perspective. You can look down and see the thoughts/clouds floating below, but you are also aware of the clear sky that exists above all those thoughts.

You can also visualize your thoughts as a river or stream. At first, you may be caught in the stream's flow. As you practice, it's as though you are stepping out of the stream onto a green, grassy bank. You can rest on the bank and allow the thoughts to flow by without getting carried away. This connects to a beautiful Buddhist saying: "When you see the river, you are out of the river."

Tips

- If you are not used to watching your thoughts, you probably don't realize how many automatic thoughts are going on all the time. The first time you do this practice, you may be shocked to find out how many thoughts are bouncing around inside your head. Remember, this is normal. Awareness is the first step toward quieting the mind.

  Research has shown that the simple act of labeling thoughts and emotions integrates the right and left hemispheres of our brain to help us feel calmer.[26]

- Everyone who tries this practice is going to feel frustrated at some point. When you sense frustration in your group, share some examples of this critical inner voice and then provide examples of a kinder voice.

Inner Critic

- "My mind is crazy."
- "If I have to sit still for another minute, I'm going to scream."
- "I can't believe I'm still thinking about that stupid thing that happened yesterday. Why can't I let it go?"
- "I'm no good at this."

Kinder Alternative

- "Everyone has crazy thoughts sometimes."
- "This is something new. It's normal to feel uncomfortable at first."
- "It's interesting that my brain can jump to so many different places in such a short amount of time!"

Or, share this quote with your group:

"If we practice mindfulness with judgment, we are growing judgment. If we practice with frustration, we are growing frustration.... Mindfulness isn't just about paying attention. It's about how we pay attention. True mindfulness involves an attitude of kindness and curiosity."

SHAUNA SHAPIRO, *GOOD MORNING, I LOVE YOU*

4.3. NAME IT TO TAME IT

Good for:

- Coping with difficult thoughts and emotions
- Calming an active or anxious mind
- Attaining perspective and balance

Introduction

This practice moves beyond observing thoughts, described in the previous practice, to focus on noticing and labeling emotions as they are happening. Your emotions, thoughts, and physical sensations all offer valuable information. The practice of mindfulness can give you access to this information and help you regain a sense of control and balance in challenging situations.

How to Practice

- Draw your awareness within. Notice the sensations of breathing.

- As you take a few deep breaths, relax the body, and slow down the breath.

- Observe your thoughts and feelings in a nonjudgmental way.

- You may notice you have different feelings bouncing around. Focus on one feeling.

- Put what you are observing into words. For example, "I feel afraid I said the wrong thing," or "I'm anxious about my appointment next week," or "This feels silly." Try to stay neutral and report on what is happening without getting carried away.

- See if you can identify where you feel this emotion in your body. Is it a sinking feeling in your gut? Or is your jaw clenched?

- After you've named what's happening inside, take a few deep breaths, let it go, and return to observing.

- Continue doing an inventory of all the feelings inside. There's no rush. Take your time and investigate each one—one at a time.

- If you notice you've gotten lost in your thoughts, it's great that you noticed it. Now you can name the thought and return to observing.

Variations

If it feels appropriate for your group, you may include these questions: "Does the emotion or its intensity fit the facts? Is there another possible perspective?" By questioning our thoughts, we open our minds to other possibilities.

Another similar practice is R.A.I.N. taught by Tara Brach,[27] author of *Radical Compassion*. See the Resources section at the end of this book to explore other variations of this practice.

Tips

- Blocking feelings intensifies them. Studies with cancer patients have shown that those who could understand, categorize, and label their emotions showed improved emotional coping and other physical health benefits, such as lower levels of inflammation.

- This exercise can be challenging because feelings can sometimes send us into rumination. This negative loop gets started when we add judgments like, "I should be over this by now," or "I should be more positive." Be watchful for any negativity or judgments. Don't get caught up in trying to fix your feeling. Let it be what it is.

o   With practice, you can improve your ability to find balance—even with difficult emotions. When I find myself ruminating about something, I repeat a little mantra that helps me apply acceptance and let go: "This moment is like this."

o   Share this quote with your group:

"There is a divine spark in all of us that enables us to pause and observe our feelings so that we can act with more grace and dignity. We can be conscious participants in life. Instead of life happening to us, we can move with a sense of purpose and mission."

JOHN LEWIS, *CARRY ON*

Source: "Name It to Tame It" is based on the work of Dr. Daniel Siegel.

4.4. MINDFUL LISTENING

Good for:

- Feeling more connected
- Cultivating present moment awareness

Introduction

The mindful listening practice is done in pairs, with each person taking turns being a speaker and a listener. It takes around 15–20 minutes. The focus here is on listening in a mindful way—being present to the speaker without adding any assumptions or judgments. Being a mindful listener includes being aware of the words *and* how they are delivered—the intonation of the speaker, the pace and pauses. The speaker's role is simply to share whatever they want and to give the listener something to listen to.

How to Practice

- Ask everyone in your group to pick a partner and explain that you're asking them to practice listening in a way that is different from how we usually listen.

- Explain the roles to the group, "There will be a listener and a speaker. We'll do two rounds so you can experience both roles."

  Listener

  - Listen, giving your full attention to the speaker.

  - You may not speak or ask questions during these three minutes.

  - You may acknowledge with facial expressions, or a nod.

- Try not to over-acknowledge.
- If the speaker runs out of things to say, give them the space for silence and be available to listen when they speak again.
- Listen for "What is true for this person at this moment in time?" Witness it; receive it unconditionally, simply to know.
- You can be practicing mindfulness, presence, and compassion. Pay attention to the effect this has on the other person. Do you notice any changes in their body language or tone of voice?

Speaker

- This is your monologue.
- You have three minutes, and you can say whatever you want.
- If you run out of things to say, that's fine. Just be silent and speak again when you have something to say.
- You can use the time in whatever ways you want. Know that whenever you are ready to speak, there is a person ready to listen to you.

- Then use a timer, allowing three minutes for the first round, three minutes for a second round with roles reversed, and three minutes at the end for the pairs to share with each other a little about their experience.

Topics for Monologue

- What are you feeling right now?
- What is something that happened today that you want to talk about?
- Any other topic that is meaningful to you.

- Finally, you may want to end with a group discussion about this experience of mindful listening. E.g.:

  - What did you notice about this experience as a listener? As a speaker?
  - How was it different from "normal" conversation?

Variation

What the speaker talks about doesn't really matter. Pick something easy and open-ended that is relevant to your group. For example, in a meditation practice group, possible topics include:

- Share your experience of meditation so far.
- Talk about why you are interested in meditation.

In a work or school setting, you might suggest:

- Share one project you are working on right now and include any details about what makes it interesting or challenging for you.

Tips

- Many speakers feel self-conscious during this exercise. It's unusual to have time and space to say whatever you want. Remind them that there's no right or wrong. This is yet another opportunity to practice being nonjudgmental of yourself.
- It can be hard for listeners to stay silent and not respond to what is being said. It takes awareness and some effort to stop our automatic way of responding.
- Complement this practice with the poem "Everything Has a Deep Dream" by Rachel Naomi Remen.

"The most basic and powerful way to connect to another person is to listen. Just listen. Perhaps the most important thing we ever give each other is our attention."

RACHEL NAOMI REMEN

Section 5:
Compassion Practices

When I was first learning about meditation and mindfulness, I received a lot of instruction about focus, attention, awareness, and the mind. Even the concepts of curiosity or nonjudgment were presented as neutral or objective players in the act of inner awareness.

Perhaps it was my own stereotype of the austere monk sitting for hours in silence that shaped this perception, but I've since discovered how incomplete that view is. Compassion, kindness, acceptance, care, generosity, and love are equally important qualities to develop—without which we cannot arrive at true wisdom, insight, or presence.

> "Love and compassion are necessities,
> not luxuries. Without them,
> humanity cannot survive."
>
> **THE DALAI LAMA**

These days, compassion is starting to get its due. The wave of scientific interest in mindfulness has expanded to include a focus on compassion research, which has shown powerful impacts for both physical and mental well-being. Practices that help you embody compassion—even for just seven minutes[28]—have been shown to boost positive feelings and a sense of social connection, and increase relaxation and immune function.

A team of researchers led by Barbara Fredrickson at the University of North Carolina found that "participants who invested an hour or so each week practicing compassion meditation enhanced a wide range of positive emotions in a wide range of situations, especially when interacting with others. Loving-kindness appears to be one positive emotion induction that keeps on giving, long after the identifiable 'event' of meditation practice."[29]

The practices shared in this section provide a range of approaches that will grow feelings of compassion and kindness toward oneself and others—and prime us to act with greater compassion. They can be used to build social connection within a group or to support individual well-being.

5.1. LOVING-KINDNESS (METTA)

Good for:

o Increasing feelings of connection
o Connecting to positive emotions

Introduction

Loving-Kindness practice involves directing your emotions toward warm and tender feelings in an open-hearted way. There are many variations, but, in general, during a loving-kindness practice you will generate kind intentions toward loved ones, yourself, and others.

This practice acknowledges our common humanity—that we all share a desire for well-being—and creates greater awareness and connection with others. It is also known as Metta Meditation and has been practiced in some form for 3,000 years in many East Asia traditions including Jainism, Hinduism, and Buddhism.

How to Practice

o Sit in a comfortable, relaxed way.

o Take two or three deep breaths at your own pace. Let the exhale be long and slow.

o Set aside any thoughts. You can pick them back up again after this practice.

o Bring to mind someone you care about. This could be a family member, friend, teacher, or even a pet. Picture this friend or loved one. Perhaps imagine being with them or think of a favorite memory of them.

- As you think of this person, notice how you feel. Notice any positive thoughts, feelings of gratitude, affection, or warmth.

- Now, you will repeat a few phrases in your mind to connect to your feelings of care for this friend or loved one. In your mind, silently repeat, *"May you be safe and happy. May you know peace and ease."*

- Shift your focus to yourself. Send yourself this same loving-kindness. Internally repeat the phrases, *"May I be safe and happy. May I know peace and ease."*

- Next, visualize someone you feel neutral about—a person you neither like nor dislike. This could be someone who lives on your street, the checker at your grocery store, or anyone that you casually know. Direct loving-kindness toward this person, silently repeating, *"May you be safe and happy. May you know peace and ease."*

- Now, think of someone you are having difficulties with, or with whom you are experiencing some conflict. Repeat your phrase of loving-kindness toward this person. *"May you be safe and happy. May you know peace and ease."*

- Finally, expand your feelings of loving-kindness toward everyone universally: *"May all beings everywhere be safe and happy. May all beings know peace and ease."*

- To end the practice, bring awareness back to your breath and into your body. Notice any effects this practice has had on your state of mind and body. Stay with any thoughts and feelings of loving-kindness that this meditation has created for you.

- Allow your body and mind to rest in the natural rhythm of breath. Thank you.

Variations

You can create your own phrases that feel natural and comfortable for you. Here are some examples:

- *May you be safe and happy. May you know peace and ease.*

- *May you be free from suffering. May you know peace and joy.*

- *May you be safe, healthy, happy, and at ease.*

- *May you be happy. May you be free from suffering. May you know peace.*

- *May you be safe. May you be peaceful. May you feel love.*

- *May you be well. May you be happy. May you be free from suffering.*

- *May you be at ease—safe and protected. May you be at peace—filled with loving-kindness.*

Rather than provide phrases for your group, you can ask questions and allow each person to generate their own version of loving-kindness. For example, you can say:

- Now, think of a wish to connect to your feelings of care for this friend or loved one. In your mind, ask yourself, "From the depths of my heart, what is it that I truly wish for this person?"

- Let your answer surface. It might be joy, meaning, safety, happiness, love, connection, or something else. Send your wish out to this person.

- Shift your focus to yourself and ask the question, "From the depths of my heart, what is it that I truly wish for myself?" Again, notice what answer comes up and send that wish to yourself.

- Finally, expand your good wishes towards everyone. Consider the question, "From the depths of my heart,

what is it that I truly wish for the people in my life?"
Again, notice what answer comes up for you. Extend
this good will out to all beings.

Tips

o For some people, this practice can evoke strong
emotions, even tears, as they think about a loved one.
You can normalize this experience by saying something
like, "it's natural and okay for this practice to evoke
strong feelings." For others, the first experience with
this practice may feel neutral. Someone might say,
"I didn't feel anything." Reassure them that this is
also normal. Repeating the phrases and holding the
intention of loving-kindness doesn't have to involve any
specific sensations. It's still having an effect.

o During practice, allow any positive feelings you do
experience to grow as you repeat the phrases—feeling
the sensations in your body. Focusing on physical
sensations creates a direct knowing that integrates the
experience more completely than a purely intellectual
approach.

o With each repetition of the phrases, you are choosing
to be kind instead of critical, but there's no need to
be fake or false. You can send people loving-kindness
without loving everything about them. In this practice,
you attempt to connect to the common humanity that
we all share, despite our differences.

o Complement this practice with the poem "Safety Net"
by Rosemerry Wahtola Trommer.

5.2. FIND A COMPASSIONATE IMAGE

Good for:
- Increasing positive emotions
- Reducing stress

Introduction

This practice asks each person to use their imagination to come up with an image of compassion that is meaningful to them. The image is used to connect to feelings of compassion and engage the whole body.

How to Practice

- Sit comfortably and close your eyes.

- What comes to mind for you when you think of something or someone that represents wisdom, strength, acceptance, love, nurturance, or caring? It might be an image of a wise person you deeply respect, or a religious figure or symbol that represents compassion to you. Or it might be an image from nature, like the expansive, deep, blue ocean, a firmly rooted tree with thick foliage, or the sun shining its light and warmth on all beings.

- Choose your own compassionate image and bring it to mind.

- Imagine yourself in the presence of this source of compassion, as the recipient of its compassion.

- Feel that in this presence you can be completely yourself. There is no judgment, only total acceptance. Allow yourself to rest in the feeling of unconditional compassion and acceptance.

- Imagine that this presence of compassion awakens your own source of strength, wisdom, courage, and compassion.

- Bring awareness to the area of your heart. Imagine filling up with compassion. As your chest expands, so does your own strength, wisdom, courage, and compassion.

- Think of a difficulty you have experienced this week and send yourself compassion, kindness, acceptance, and understanding. For several breaths, rest in the warmth of that feeling.

- Bring awareness back to your breath. Noticing any effects this practice of compassion has had on your state of mind and body.

Variation

This practice is similar to Gazing (3.2), where you focus on an external image as a stabilizing object of focus. It's possible to find and use a physical image or object that represents compassion, instead of creating an image in your mind.

Tips

- When using imagery, it's helpful to remind people that there is no right or wrong. For some people, conjuring up a vivid image helps them stay focused. Other people may get too involved, trying to get every detail "right," in which case it's better to focus on a simple, holistic image. Then there may be people who get caught up in decision paralysis and can't decide what image to choose. Again, remind them that there's no right or wrong, and there's no harm in trying something. If they find themselves judging or evaluating their choice, encourage them to let go of thinking as much as possible and pick one image to focus on.

○ Visualization allows you to go to a place without words and conceptual thinking. Creating and embodying an image can help us move from discursive thinking to experiential being. Experiment and see if you can get absorbed with the senses and your direct experience.

Source: Hanson, M. L. *Cultivating Compassion: Four Science-Backed Strategies for Strengthening Compassion.* Stanford University, CCARE, 2013.

5.3. COMPASSION FOR A LOVED ONE

Good for:

○ Enhancing social connections

○ Increasing positive emotions, including empathy and self-compassion

Introduction

You may be asking, "How is compassion different from loving-kindness?" A very good question! Loving-kindness is something you can feel under any circumstance. Compassion is more specific—something you feel in the face of suffering. It can include both feelings of concern (empathy) and a motivation to see suffering relieved.

Compassion can be more challenging than loving-kindness— because it requires us to face suffering. Compassion is a natural instinct that everyone has, and it's also a skill you can grow and strengthen.

In this practice, you will choose a specific friend or loved one to help you generate thoughts and feelings of compassion. Who you choose is not as important as your intention to cultivate this feeling within yourself.

How to Practice

○ Find a comfortable position and take a few deep breaths.

○ Allow the breath to settle into its own natural rhythm and pace. For a few moments, just focus on your breath. Let yourself experience and be aware of the sensations of breathing.

- Choose a friend or loved one and bring them to mind. Remember or imagine a time when this loved one was suffering in some way. Maybe they were sick or in pain, maybe they were experiencing disappointment or loss, maybe they were in a confusing or difficult situation. Recall that specific time.

- Notice how you feel. You may feel sad or upset. Or you may notice feelings of warmth or tenderness toward your friend or loved one. Notice any urges to comfort or support this friend or loved one.

- Choosing to focus your attention on feelings of tenderness or the desire to help, silently repeat the following phrases for your friend or loved one: "*May you be free from suffering. May you know peace.*"

- Connect this to your breath. As you exhale, send out your compassionate feelings of care and support for your friend: "*May you be free from suffering. May you know peace.*"

- Next, bring one hand to the center of your chest, the area around your physical heart. Notice how this area gently expands and fills as you breathe in, and relaxes and releases as you breathe out.

- As you're breathing out, imagine extending a warmth or a beam of light from the center of your heart. This warmth or light carries all your thoughts and feelings of compassion. Imagine this warmth or light touching your friend, bringing them peace and happiness. And once again silently repeat, "*May you be free from suffering. May you know peace.*"

- Bring awareness back to your breath. Notice and stay with any thoughts and feelings of compassion that this meditation has created. And in the last few moments, simply allow your body and mind to rest in the natural rhythm of the breath. Thank you.

Variation

In preparation for leading this exercise, you might invite your group to first remember a personal experience of compassion. For example, "Take a moment to think, when have you experienced compassion being given or received? Bring this moment to mind and notice how it makes you feel. Do you feel an expansion in your chest? Or warmth in your cheeks? A smile on your face? There's no right or wrong way to feel. Close your eyes and notice how it feels in your body. See if you can connect with any physical feelings of compassion."

Tips

- This meditation can evoke strong feelings, mixed emotions, or no particular feelings or emotions at all, and that's okay. The important point is to develop the intention to cultivate an attitude of compassion. Whatever feelings or emotions arise, acknowledge that direct experience. Then, continue to focus on the images, words, and ideas in this practice.

- Directing your mind in this way allows your mind and heart to become more aligned with the qualities of compassion and loving-kindness.

Source: This exercise is adapted from the CCT™ curriculum developed at Stanford University Center for Compassion and Altruism Research and Education (CCARE).

EMBODYING EMOTIONS

Sometimes our *thoughts* influence our *bodies*. For example, thinking about something that makes you angry can raise your blood pressure, or cause tension in your jaw, or a tightness in your stomach.

It works the other way around, too! Changes in your *body* can change how you *think or feel*. For example, it's well-documented that regular exercise can reduce depression.[30]

Many of the practices in this book emphasize *embodiment*—the felt sense of thoughts and feelings in the physical body. It's useful to tune in to what's going on inside your body to get clues about what you or others are feeling and to increase connection with yourself and others.

The experience of empathy is especially interesting in this regard. Without even thinking about it, we use our bodies to mimic and understand what other people are feeling. For example, when someone smiles at you, do you smile back? The smile on your face triggers your awareness that the smiling person is feeling good.

Perhaps the most interesting evidence of this body/mind connection comes from a 2011 study of people who received Botox injections to remove wrinkles in their face, but which also inhibit a person's ability to move their facial muscles. Researchers found that the inability to mirror the faces of others resulted in a reduced ability to perceive the emotions of others, effectively causing emotional blindness.[31]

5.4. SELF-COMPASSION

Good for:

- Increasing feelings of connection
- Reducing stress and self-criticism

Introduction

This practice is designed to stretch us a little bit—to call up some personal difficulty and apply self-compassion. Through in-depth research, Dr. Kristin Neff has identified that self-compassion has three key elements—mindfulness, common humanity, and self-kindness—and this practice touches on all three.

How to Practice

- Start by drawing your awareness within. Notice the breath.

- First, think of a good friend or loved one—someone you care deeply about. Connect to your feelings of warmth, care, and compassion for this person. Repeat the phrases, "May you be free from suffering. May you know peace and ease."

- Now, turn your feelings of warmth, care, and concern to yourself. Bring to mind something that is creating some stress, pain, or suffering for you this week. Notice how you feel when you think about this.

- Acknowledge what you are experiencing. For example, you might say to yourself, "This is really hard right now. This is stress. This is a moment of suffering."

- Consider the possibility that this difficulty does not isolate you from others but is part of the experience of being human. You might repeat one of these phrases, "It's normal to feel this way. Many people are going through similar struggles."

- o Amid all the feelings that may come up, notice any feelings of tenderness, warmth, and concern. Be supportive and encouraging to yourself. For example, "May I be kind to myself in this moment. There's nothing wrong with me. May I be patient. May I learn not to be so hard on myself."

- o Maybe place a hand over your heart as you send loving-kindness and compassion to yourself. Repeat the phrases, "May I be free from suffering. May I know peace and ease."

- o Take a deep breath, absorbing that experience.

- o And when you're ready, open your eyes and come back to the room.

Variation

If it's appropriate for your group, you can extend this practice of self-compassion into some group appreciation. For example:

- o Take a moment to look around and see the compassion and kindness that's present within our group. The safety and support that is here.

- o As a way to offer recognition to each other, I invite you to find a physical gesture, maybe a bow or a hand on your heart, as you send your wish to this group: "May you be free from suffering. May you have access to your inner resources to navigate life with greater ease. May you feel loved and accepted just as you are. May you know that you belong. And may you be at peace."

- Take a moment and receive and feel those good wishes coming back to you now. Breathe those in and feel the support and warmth of this community.

Tips

- You may want to suggest that people pick a difficulty or challenge that feels manageable to work with. Start small at first.

- Many people find that having compassion for themselves can be harder than having compassion for others. This is understandable. As Stanford psychologist Dr. Kelly McGonigal writes, "We're wired to be critical of ourselves and compassionate toward others because we want to be accepted by the group. We must learn to turn our innate natural compassion instinct toward ourselves." Self-compassion gets easier with practice!

- Complement this practice with the poem "Love After Love" by Derek Walcott. Or, share this quote with your group:

"Having compassion for yourself
means that you honor and accept
your humanness. Things will not always
go the way you want them to.
You will encounter frustrations, losses
will occur, you will make mistakes,
bump up against your limitations, fall
short of your ideals.

This is the human condition, a reality
shared by all of us. The more you open
your heart to this reality instead of
constantly fighting against it, the more

you will be able to feel compassion
for yourself and all your fellow humans
in the experience of life."

DR. KRISTIN NEFF[32]

COMPASSION FOR THE INNER CRITIC

Perhaps the biggest obstacle to self-compassion is the inner critic. We all have an inner critic that is monitoring and judging our actions, and sending negative messages like, "You should have... Why didn't you...?" We often think these messages are somehow going to motivate us to be "better" or protect us from doing something "wrong," but research shows this isn't true. Self-compassion, not self-criticism, creates resilience and the courage to continue after mistakes, setbacks, and failures.

When working with a group, ask people to notice inner judgments, and try having compassion for the self-critic. Dr. Kristin Neff suggests talking back to your inner critic, saying something like, "I appreciate what you're trying to do for me. Thanks for your efforts. I'm going to try something different: Kindness."

With practice, we can learn to motivate ourselves with compassion instead of criticism. In place of self-blaming messages such as "What's wrong with me?", self-compassion asks, "What can I learn? How can I grow?"

"Maybe we need to make some changes—
not because we are inadequate—but because
we love ourselves and we don't want to suffer.
'I believe in you, and I know you can do it.'
If we love and care about ourselves, we are
going to want to do everything we can to
reach our full potential."

DR. KRISTIN NEFF,
THE SELF-ACCEPTANCE PROJECT

"You have peace
when you make it
with yourself."

MITCH ALBOM

5.5. COMPASSIONATE TOUCH

Good for:

- When you only have a minute or two
- Lowering heart rate and blood pressure
- Strengthening the immune system
- Increasing feelings of trust, safety, and (you guessed it!) compassion

Introduction

Many of the practices in this book explore how the physical body influences mental and emotional states. For example, slowing down your breathing can calm your mind. So it's probably no surprise that physical touch—a hug, a pat on the back, or even petting a dog—has well-documented health benefits. Touch activates our caregiving systems.

It might sound silly, but you can get all these benefits by hugging yourself! When you are under stress, all you need to do is apply gentle touch to yourself with the intent to soothe.

How to Practice

There are different physical gestures that can trigger a shift to compassion. Take a couple deep breaths as you try one of these:

(1) Put your hand on your heart, or both hands over the heart.

(2) Cross your arms and give yourself a gentle squeeze.

(3) Cross your arms and put your hands at the top of your shoulders, then move your hands from your shoulders down to your elbows. Repeat.

Feel yourself both as the giver and receiver of compassion.

Variation

You can invite people to silently say an affirmation at the same time. For example:

- "I am okay."
- "I am strong."
- "I am supported."

Tip

- When life is stressful and there is a lot going on, it's easy to get disconnected or caught up in negative feelings. Compassion may not change your situation, but it might change how you feel about it.

5.6. JUST LIKE ME

Good for:

- ○ Increasing feelings of connection
- ○ Reducing stress and feelings of social pressure

Introduction

This practice can be done as a whole group or in pairs. As the leader, you'll be guiding people to consider different phrases that reflect the ways we are all the same. This recognition of our common humanity is a key component to accessing compassion for ourselves and others.

Before you begin, orient the group. Let them know that you'll be sharing phrases for them to reflect upon and tell them about how much time the practice will last. It's normal for people to feel resistance, emotions, or mental chatter. Remind them that those are all natural experiences, to be aware of the thoughts, and then to let them go. This is a practice of returning to common humanity over and over again.

How to Practice

- ○ If you are doing this meditation in pairs, sit facing your partner and meet their gaze. If not, close your eyes and draw someone to mind—a friend, a coworker, or perhaps someone you are having some difficulty with right now.

- ○ Find an anchor. This could be awareness of your breath, your feet resting on the floor, or your hands resting on your legs. Know that you are safe and supported in this practice.

- Bring your awareness to the person in front of you, either the person you have in your mind or the one actually sitting across from you.
- Silently repeat these phrases while looking at your partner.
  - "This person has a body and a mind, just like me."
  - "This person has feelings, thoughts, and emotions, just like me."
  - "This person has experienced suffering at some point in their life, just like me."
- Take a breath and feel the truth of those statements.
  - "Just like me, at some point in their life, this person has been angry."
  - "Just like me, this person has at times felt scared or afraid."
  - "Just like me, this person has been deeply disappointed and sad."
  - "Just like me, this person wants to feel safe and protected."
  - "Just like me, this person wants to feel loved and accepted, just as they are."
  - "Just like me, this person wants to be happy and be at peace."
- To complete the practice, turn this awareness of common humanity into a wish for well-being for your partner: "May you feel safe and protected, loved and accepted, just as you are. May you be happy. And may you be at peace."

- Expand this wish to include your whole group and yourself: "May we all feel safe and protected, loved and accepted, just as we are. May we all be happy and at peace."

- Reconnect with your anchor. Feel your breath and your body. Slowly transition back to an awareness of the room and the space around you. Thank your partner for doing this practice with you.

Variation

This practice is especially effective with an online group that meets using video. Ask that people use "gallery view" so they can see everyone's face. As you repeat each phrase, invite people to first focus on one face, and then shift focus to a new face with each new phrase.

Tips

- Pause and allow time between each phrase as you read it aloud.

- Feel free to adjust the phrases provided to phrases that are comfortable for you and appropriate for your group.

- After we've had a profound or deep experience, it's beneficial to name it as a way of helping to integrate the experience. You might suggest that people give a name to their experience at the end of this practice: "Find a few words for what you're taking with you from this experience and write them down."

Source: This practice is inspired by Mirabai Bush, founding director of The Center for Contemplative Mind.

"Our human compassion binds us the one to the other—not in pity or patronizingly, but as human beings who have learnt how to turn our common suffering into hope for the future."

NELSON MANDELA

5.7. TONGLEN

Good for:

- o Growing compassion
- o Developing emotional balance and strength

Introduction

Tonglen is a Tibetan word that means "giving and receiving." This is a Buddhist practice that goes right to the core of compassion. To understand Tonglen, you must first understand the definition of compassion.

> *Compassion* is a sense of concern that we have when we are confronted with suffering and feel motivated to see that suffering relieved.

Compassion includes awareness, empathy, and action—and the practice of Tonglen touches on all three. In this practice, we accept suffering (awareness) and at the same time seek to transform it with empathy and action.

How to Practice

- o Set an intention to cultivate compassion in yourself. This requires the willingness to accept difficulties or suffering and look them head on. Acknowledge the innate courage, strength, and compassion that we all have and can develop with practice.
- o Bring to mind some small suffering in your life.

  - o Inhale, noticing your ability to hold and accept the reality of that suffering.

  - o Exhale, with the wish to give comfort and send relief or healing to yourself.

- Gradually expand your awareness to include others who may be experiencing a similar difficulty, loss, or pain in their lives.
  - Inhale, imagining that you can take away some of that suffering.
  - Exhale, and imagine transforming suffering into healing, well-being, or peace.
- If you like, you can expand your awareness to include all beings.
  - Inhale, acknowledging there is pain and suffering in the world.
  - Exhale, with the intention to help others.
- You might imagine sending out warmth from your heart. Or imagine suffering as a dark cloud. You can draw in some of that darkness and dissolve it in the radiant light in your heart. On the out-breath, send out the bright healing energy from your heart.
- To close the practice, check in with your body. Do you notice any effects of the practice on how you feel?

Variations

The script above starts with choosing a specific personal suffering and expanding the practice from there. You may choose other starting points. For example, this practice can be done for someone specific that you know who is experiencing some difficulty. Or you may take a more universal approach and begin this practice with an intent to relieve suffering in the world on a more global level.

There are many lessons embedded in this practice—one of them is the lesson that we can choose our thoughts. Just as our breath changes from inhale to exhale, our thoughts can change, too. With this in mind, you can practice Tonglen with two colors. Inhale blue and exhale yellow. Or inhale magenta and exhale electric green. You can pick any two colors you want. The point of this practice is to notice that we have an ability to change our thoughts and have some degree of control over our thoughts. Powerful stuff!

Tips

- In nearly every description of Tonglen that I've read, people emphasize the difficulty of the practice. It's *"not for beginners,"* they'll say. "No one wants to breathe in pain." I'm not sure I agree. Imagine that you come upon someone in the road with a broken arm. How would you try to help them? Would you help relieve their pain by breaking your own arm, or would you find a brace or a sling to help hold and ease their pain and try to get them to a hospital? Tonglen is no different. You are not inhaling suffering to bring it onto yourself, but to hold it with an intent to bring comfort and ease.

- We often try to avoid, ignore, or deny difficulties, so sitting and facing the reality of difficulty, pain, or suffering takes some courage. Invite your group to consider how this practice develops their own sources of courage and strength.

- Tonglen is one way of practicing *radical acceptance*, the psychological skill of accepting things that are outside our control—even difficulties and discomforts— without judgement. My favorite phrase of acceptance is "this moment is like this." If contemplating pain or suffering feels overwhelming, try repeating this phrase.

- One image that can be helpful in this practice is to imagine a huge headlight at the center of your chest shining out into the night. See yourself as a car on a dark road. With each inhale, move through the darkness; and with each exhale, radiate light that cuts through the darkness, allowing you to see the road ahead. An image of a lighthouse, steady and strong, may also be useful.

o Someone in your group may ask, "Is sending healing thoughts really an action?" This is debatable, but what we do know is that this practice primes us to view the world with greater compassion. Your intentions will have impact not just during the time that you practice, but beyond.

o Acts of compassion often don't involve us "fixing" something for someone else, but instead require that we believe in them and their ability to heal. Sending them strength, knowing that they have the inner resources to meet their challenge, is an empowering point of view to take.

o Share this quote with your group:

> "Compassion in action is paradoxical and mysterious.... It accepts that everything is happening exactly as it should, and it works with a full-hearted commitment to change.... It intends to eliminate suffering, knowing that suffering is limitless."[33]
>
> **RAM DASS**

Closing

The practices outlined here are designed to be accessible for beginners and provide an entry point to a direct experience of the benefits of meditation, mindfulness, and compassion, including:

- Reducing stress and promoting healing
- Creating a sense of calm and well-being
- Sharpening attention and focusing the mind
- Opening to greater creativity and connection
- Bringing perspective and self-acceptance
- Growing compassion and fostering spiritual development

Yet, this book only scratches the surface. If you are interested in facilitating practices with groups, you surely already know that meditation is a path that can lead to deep places of healing, connection, and consciousness.

I hope that your interest in spreading the benefits of group practice will blossom and grow. And, that this book will give you confidence and inspiration to find your own style and make this your own.

As you continue on your journey, may you find additional resources and teachers to help you deepen your personal practice, and may you find ways to share what you learn with others.

"Mindfulness, self-compassion, and the practices that emerge from them help free us from the prison of isolation and the delusion of separation. These practices open our minds, awaken our hearts, and deepen our sense of connection with ourselves, each other, and our world. We begin to realize that we are never just practicing for ourselves. Transforming ourselves creates echoes in the universe. As we heal ourselves, we heal each other, and our world."

SHAUNA SHAPIRO,
GOOD MORNING, I LOVE YOU

Thank you for reading this book!

If you found this book helpful, inspiring, or even
just thought-provoking, please take a moment
to leave a quick review wherever you purchased it.
Your insights not only help me improve,
but also help other readers discover the book.

★ ★ ★ ★ ★

You can also share your thoughts
directly with me online.

holdingspaceguide.com

Acknowledgments

Heartfelt thanks to the many friends, family, and colleagues who read drafts of this book and offered feedback; Sarah Miller, Joshua Salesin, Monica Hanson, Barbara Price, Rob McNeil, Sharon Schneeberger, Belinda Haan, Julia Townsend, Nancy Goldman, and Howard Rappaport for the gifts of your time and insight.

Special mention goes to Sarah Miller for believing in this book from the very beginning and being my first reader, coach, cheerleader, and friend. You are the natural writer that I aspire to be.

This book would not exist without the support of Belinda Haan, my compassion sister. I am so grateful for your wise encouragement and for lighting my path as a new author. You gave me the confidence to keep going through moments of uncertainty.

To my professional editors, Crystal Nero and Melissa McDaniel, much appreciation to you for bringing clarity and polish to the text. Appreciation also goes to Silke Spingies for the beautiful cover and layout of this book.

I am grateful for the diverse teachers and communities that support me:

I could never adequately convey my appreciation for Monica Hanson, my first teacher in compassion cultivation at Stanford CCARE as well as a co-founder of the Applied Compassion Training (ACT). Your care and kind attention have supported my growth as an ambassador of compassion.

I am grateful to you for reading the manuscript and providing insightful feedback, and for your dear friendship.

Thank you to two other Stanford ACT directors, Neelama Eyers and Robert Cusick. My time in ACT is what led to this project. In addition, my ACT colleagues continue to provide inspiration, encouragement, and resources—including Belinda Haan, Barbara Price, Nancy Goldman, Theresa Meikle, Catherine Schweikert, Katie Huey, Cindy Gum, Jeff Jacobs, Kristine Claghorn, Suzanne McCormac, Helene Creager, and a special shout out to the class of '22.

Many others contributed their personal and professional experience. Both knowingly and unknowingly, Divya Zuccaro, Marc Morozumi, and Eric Gustafson have inspired me with their teaching and writings.

I would like to recognize the WomenCARE staff and volunteers for their compassion and generosity, and especially for creating a community filled with genuine acceptance and support. Special shout outs to LaVerne Coleman, Paula Sims, and Roberta Hill for their leadership.

Thank you from the bottom of my heart to the members of the WomenCARE meditation circle (past, present, and future), including Jacquie, Roberta, Judy, Anna, Mohini, Bonnie, Luann, Pat, Beth, Pamela, Diana, Stephanie, Melody, Carolyn, and more.

The Redwood Rx program at Mountain Parks Foundation, led by Brenda Holmes, has been instrumental in opening up new avenues for my teaching. I also want to acknowledge the inspiring community of instructors within the program, especially Kai Siedenburg, who generously shared her practices with me.

I am grateful for the friends who supported me through my writing struggles and progress, Lisa, Stacia, Aria, Polly,

Carolyn, Chithra, Christie, Sorab, Anne, Sally, Sara, Margaret, Nandu, Bess, Dina, Ali, Tam, Regina, and Katherine.

The Integral Yoga San Francisco Institute has also been a source of wisdom, teaching, and community. Thank you Swami Ramananda and Diana Meltsner for your teaching and guidance in meditation, and Rich Panico for adding in the perspective of early Buddhism.

I am most fortunate to have Radha Vignola as my first meditation and yoga teacher. It is her kind voice, radiant acceptance, and ongoing curiosity that have nurtured my growth as a student and teacher.

To my parents, Ken and Sharon, and my brother, Peter, for your unwavering belief in me.

And finally, thank you most of all to Joshua, who makes me laugh and keeps me going when I feel stuck. You remind me that life is a creative process to be discovered and appreciated.

In memory of three deeply creative people who I am honored to have known and who continue to inspire my days, Tana Butler, Tripura Anand, and Kristin Smith Westbrook.

Resources

Meditation & Mindfulness

Brach, Tara. "How to Start a Mindfulness Meditation Group." www.tarabrach.com/starting-meditation-group.

Brach, Tara. "RAIN: Recognize, Allow, Investigate, Nurture." January 31, 2024. www.tarabrach.com/rain.

The Greater Good Science Center. "Greater Good in Action." ggia.berkeley.edu.

Kornfield, Jack. *Meditation for Beginners*. Sounds True, 2010.

Siegel, Daniel J. *Mindsight: The New Science of Personal Transformation*. Random House Publishing Group, 2010.

Tan, Chade-Meng, et al. *Search Inside Yourself: The Unexpected Path to Achieving Success, Happiness (and World Peace)*. HarperOne, 2014.

"YoMIND." Vimeo. vimeo.com/yomind.

Yongey Mingyur, and Helen Tworkov. *In Love with the World: A Monk's Journey Through the Bardos of Living and Dying*. Random House, 2021.

Compassion

McGonigal, Kelly. *The Science of Compassion: A Modern Approach for Cultivating Empathy, Love, and Connection*. Sounds True, 2016.

Neff, Kristin. *Self-Compassion*. William Morrow, 2011.

Shapiro, Shauna L. *Good Morning, I Love You: Mindfulness and Self-Compassion Practices to Rewire Your Brain for Calm, Clarity and Joy*. Sounds True, 2022.

Health & Healing

Bonior, Andrea. *Detox Your Thoughts: Quit Negative Self-Talk for Good and Discover the Life You've Always Wanted*. Chronicle Books, 2021.

Devine, Megan. *It's OK That You're NOT OK: Meeting Grief and Loss in a Culture That Doesn't Understand*. Sounds True, 2018.

Kabat-Zinn, Jon. *Mindfulness Meditation for Pain Relief: Practices to Reclaim Your Body and Your Life*. Sounds True, 2023.

Nhất Hạnh, Thich, and Annabel Laity. *The Blooming of a Lotus: Guided Meditation Exercises for Healing and Transformation*. Beacon Press, 1993.

Sandberg, Sheryl, and Adam M. Grant. *Option B: Facing Adversity, Building Resilience, and Finding Joy*. WH Allen, an Imprint of Ebury Publishing, 2019.

Stuntz, Elizabeth Cohn, and Marsha Linehan. *Coping with Cancer: DBT Skills to Manage Your Emotions—and Balance Uncertainty with Hope*. The Guilford Press, 2021.

Westbrook, Kristin Smith. *The Luckiest Unlucky Person I Know: A Practical Memoir*. New Degree Press, 2023.

Williams, J. Mark G., et al. *The Mindful Way through Depression: Freeing Yourself from Chronic Unhappiness*. Sounds True, 2008.

Facilitation

Arlin Cuncic, MA. "7 Active Listening Techniques to Practice in Your Daily Conversations." Verywell Mind. February 12, 2024. www.verywellmind.com/what-is-active-listening-3024343.

The Circle Way. "The Circle Way." www.thecircleway.net.

Crane, Rebecca S., et al. *Manual of the Mindfulness-Based Interventions Teaching Assessment Criteria*. Centre for Mindfulness Research and Practice, Bangor University, Third Version: 2021.

Simply Psychology. "Active Listening: Definition, Skills, & Benefits." December 20, 2023. www.simplypsychology.org/active-listening-definition-skills-benefits.html.

Poetry

Easwaran, Eknath. *God Makes the Rivers to Flow: Sacred Literature of the World*. Nilgiri Press, 2003.

Goff-Maidoff, Ingrid. *What Holds Us: New and Selected Poems*. Sarah's Circle Publishing, 2011.

Hirshfield, Jane. *Ledger*. Bloodaxe Books, 2020.

Oliver, Mary. *A Thousand Mornings*. Penguin Books, 2014.

Patel, Kaveri. *An Invitation*. Kaveri Patel, 2011.

Trauma-Informed Resources

Cheetah House. "Help for Meditators in Distress." cheetahhouse.org.

Menakem, Resmaa. *My Grandmother's Hands: Racialized Trauma and the Pathway to Mending Our Hearts and Bodies*. Penguin Books, 2021.

Rice, Andrea. "A Guide to Trauma-Informed Mindfulness." PsychCentral. January 5, 2022. psychcentral.com/health/trauma-informed-mindfulness.

Spoon, Marianne. "How Meditation Can Be More Sensitive to Trauma." Greater Good. March 5, 2021. greatergood.berkeley.edu/article/item/how_meditation_can_be_more_sensitive_to_trauma.

Appendix

Here's an example of a group description and meeting outline for the one-hour meditation circle that I lead for members of WomenCARE.

WomenCARE Meditation Circle

Meeting on the first and third Fridays of each month from 11–12

The WomenCARE meditation circle is an ongoing group open to anyone who wants to learn about, and practice, meditation. Meetings provide an opportunity to learn tools from ancient traditions and modern science and identify practices that work well for you. No prior experience required.

Each meeting includes three rounds of meditation practice as well as time for members to check in and share their experiences and questions. We explore a range of meditation and mindfulness techniques known to reduce stress, stabilize the mind, and promote health and well-being.

FACILITATOR OUTLINE

Start the zoom about five minutes before 11a and welcome and greet members as they join. A typical meeting will have 4–8 people in attendance. The general flow of each meeting is:

11:00–11:05 (4–5 mins)	**Meet and Greet** Allow time for people to join. Check and see if there are any first timers and if so, find out a bit about their experience with meditation and provide extra instructions and support so that they feel comfortable.
11:05–11:12 (7–8 mins)	**Breath-Based Meditation** Introduce and lead 7–8 mins of any breath based meditation. The goal is to allow people a tangible way to arrive in the present moment.
11:12–11:25 (10–15 mins)	**Check-Ins** Invite people to share a little bit about themselves and how they are doing, if they want to. Encourage people to include any questions that they may have for the group. (Sometime people will share anxiety about an upcoming test or ask for advice from the group about dealing with something specific.) Hold the space and make sure everyone who wants to check in has a chance to speak completely—without getting cut off. You may choose to ask people to answer a question during their check-in, such as: "Do you have any requests for our meditation today? What do you get out of meditation?

Check-Ins continued...

Do you have any questions about meditation?
Do you have any questions for me?"

*Note that when there are fewer attendees, the
check in period will be shorter. You can increase
each round of meditation by 1–2 minutes to
balance out the time.*

11:25–11:35 (7–8 mins)	**Second Round of Meditation** Introduce and lead 7–8 minutes of meditation. In the second round, we explore different aspects of meditation and experiment with different techniques. If you want, you can share a poem or short reading. For example: o Discuss the practice of Tonglen and the concept that we can choose our thoughts. Then practice breathing in one color and breathing out another. o Discuss open awareness and present moment awareness and practice mindfulness meditation. o Discuss the benefits of objectivity and practice "Name It to Tame It."
11:35–11:45 (5 mins)	**Open Discussion** Give members an opportunity to share their experience with the group.

11:45–11:58 (12–13 mins)	**Compassion Meditation**

11:45–11:58
(12–13 mins)

Compassion Meditation

The third round of meditation is usually 12–13 minutes to allow members to go a little deeper.

I encourage those with a regular practice to do that during the third round.* And, I always offer up a compassion meditation for those that don't yet have a dedicated practice. Possible compassion meditations include:

o Loving-Kindness

o Tonglen

o Self-Compassion

* I've encouraged members to find their regular practice. While it's good to have a range of practices and tools to use in different situations, it's also valuable to find one practice to use consistently. When we consistently practice one thing, we get really good at it.

11:58–12:00
(2 mins)

Closure

Thank members for joining, for taking the time for self-care, and for supporting each other by participating in the group.

Remind them of the date and time of the next meeting.

Notes

Chapter 1

1 Deep gratitude goes to the teachers of the Applied Compassion Training (ACT) at Stanford's Center for Compassion and Altruism Research and Education (CCARE). For more about CCARE, visit https://ccare.stanford.edu.

2 I am also deeply grateful for the expertise and guidance from my meditation instructors at the Integral Yoga Institute of San Francisco (IYISF). For more information about their trainings, visit https://integralyogasf.org.

Chapter 2

3 Mindful Staff. "Jon Kabat-Zinn: Defining Mindfulness." Mindful. January 11, 2017.
https://www.mindful.org/jon-kabat-zinn-defining-mindfulness.

4 Derived from work of Erika Rosenberg, Ph.D.

5 Gilbert, Paul, and William Van Gordon. "Compassion as a Skill: A Comparison of Contemplative and Evolution-Based Approaches." *Mindfulness* 14, no. 10 (August 2023): 2395–2416. https://doi.org/10.1007/s12671-023-02173-w.

6 Kornfield, Jack. *Meditation for Beginners*. Sounds True, 2010, p. 14.

7 Goleman, Daniel, and Richard J. Davidson. *Altered Traits: Science Reveals How Meditation Changes Your Mind, Brain, and Body*. Avery, an Imprint of Penguin Random House LLC, 2017.

8   Witek-Janusek, L., et al. "Effect of Mindfulness-Based Stress Reduction on Immune Function, Quality of Life and Coping in Women Newly Diagnosed with Early-Stage Breast Cancer." *Brain, Behavior, and Immunity* 22, no. 6 (2008): 969–981. https://doi.org/10.1016/j.bbi.2008.01.012.

9   Goleman, Daniel, and Richard J. Davidson. *Altered Traits: Science Reveals How Meditation Changes Your Mind, Brain, and Body.* Avery, an Imprint of Penguin Random House LLC, 2017.

10 Stuntz, Elizabeth Cohn, and Marsha Linehan. *Coping with Cancer: DBT Skills to Manage Your Emotions—and Balance Uncertainty with Hope.* The Guilford Press, 2021.

11 Desbordes, Gaëlle, et al. "Effects of Mindful-Attention and Compassion Meditation Training on Amygdala Response to Emotional Stimuli in an Ordinary, Non-meditative State." *Frontiers in Human Neuroscience* 6 (2012). https://doi.org/10.3389/fnhum.2012.00292.

12 Kemper, K., Shaltout, H., Tooze, J. et al. "P05.11. Time, Touch, and Compassion: Effects on Autonomic Nervous System and Well-being." *BMC Complementary and Alternative Medicine* 12, no. Suppl 1 (2012): P371. https://doi.org/10.1186/1472-6882-12-S1-P371.

Chapter 3

13 Centers for Disease Control and Prevention. "Fast Facts: Preventing Adverse Childhood Experiences." October 8, 2024. https://www.cdc.gov/aces/about.

14 Spoon, Marianne. "How Meditation Can Be More Sensitive to Trauma." Greater Good. March 5, 2021. https://greatergood.berkeley.edu/article/item/how_meditation_can_be_more_sensitive_to_trauma.

15 Crane, Rebecca S., et al. *Manual of the Mindfulness-Based Interventions Teaching Assessment Criteria.* Centre for Mindfulness Research and Practice, Bangor University, Third Version: 2021, p. 58.

Chapter 4

16 Healing Circles Global. "Healing Circles Agreements." https://healingcirclesglobal.org/healing-circles-agreements.

17 Schweikert, Catherine W. *The Compassion Remedy.* WorldChangers Media, 2023, pp. 131-132.

18 Balban, Melis Yilmaz, et al. "Brief Structured Respiration Practices Enhance Mood and Reduce Physiological Arousal." *Cell Reports Medicine* 4, no. 1 (January 2023): 100895. https://doi.org/10.1016/j.xcrm.2022.100895.

19 Vimeo. "YoMIND." https://vimeo.com/yomind.

Chapter 5

20 Singer, Tania. "What Type of Meditation Is Best for You?" Greater Good. July 2, 2018. https://greatergood.berkeley.edu/article/item/what_type_of_meditation_is_best_for_you.

21 McGonigal, Kelly. "The Big Brain Benefits of Meditation." Yoga Journal. May 16, 2024. https://www.yogajournal.com/lifestyle/health/brain-meditation.

22 McGonigal, Kelly. "Your Brain on Meditation." Mindful. November16, 2023. https://www.mindful.org/your-brain-on-meditation.

23 Kok, B. E., K. A. Coffey, M. A. Cohn, L. I. Catalino, T. Vacharkulksemsuk, S. B. Algoe, M. Brantley, and B. L. Fredrickson. "How Positive Emotions Build Physical Health: Perceived Positive Social Connections Account for the Upward Spiral Between Positive Emotions and Vagal Tone." *Psychological Science* 24, no. 7 (2013): 1123-1132. https://doi.org/10.1177/0956797612470827.

24 Schiffmann, Erich. *Yoga: The Spirit and Practice of Moving into Stillness.* Pocket Books, 1996.

25 Stuntz, Elizabeth Cohn, and Marsha Linehan. *Coping with Cancer: DBT Skills to Manage Your Emotions—and Balance Uncertainty with Hope.* The Guilford Press, 2021. p. 24.

26 Lieberman M.D., N. I. Eisenberger, M. J. Crockett, S. M. Tom, J. H. Pfeifer, and B. M. Way. "Putting Feelings into Words: Affect Labeling Disrupts Amygdala Activity in Response to Affective Stimuli." *Psychological Science* 18, no. 5 (2007): 421–428. https://doi.org/10.1111/j.1467-9280.2007.01916.x.

27 Tara Brach. "Resources ~ Rain: Recognize, Allow, Investigate, Nurture." January 31, 2024. https://www.tarabrach.com/rain.

28 Hutcherson, Cendri A., et al. "Loving-Kindness Meditation Increases Social Connectedness." *Emotion* 8, no. 5 (October 2008): 720–724. https://doi.org/10.1037/a0013237.

29 Fredrickson, Barbara L., et al. "Open Hearts Build Lives: Positive Emotions, Induced through Loving-Kindness Meditation, Build Consequential Personal Resources." *Journal of Personality and Social Psychology* 95, no. 5 (2008): 1045–1062. https://doi.org/10.1037/a0013262.

30 Harvard Health. "Exercise Is an All-Natural Treatment to Fight Depression." February 2, 2021. https://www.health.harvard.edu/mind-and-mood/exercise-is-an-all-natural-treatment-to-fight-depression.

31 Paul, Pamela. "With Botox, Looking Good and Feeling Less." The New York Times. June 17, 2011. https://www.nytimes.com/2011/06/19/fashion/botox-reduces-the-ability-to-empathize-study-says.html.

32 Self-Compassion. "Compassion by Kristin Neff." July 9, 2024. https://self-compassion.org.

33 Omega. "Compassion in Action." https://www.eomega.org/article/compassion-in-action.

About the Author

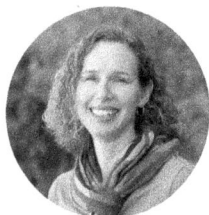

Claire Schneeberger has been teaching meditation and compassion since 2013. She is certified as a meditation teacher through the Integral Yoga Institute of San Francisco and as an ambassador of compassion through Stanford's Center for Compassion and Altruism Research and Education (CCARE).

She facilitates workshops and ongoing groups to support well-being in workplaces and community spaces, including in her beloved state parks near her home in Santa Cruz, CA. With a professional background in learning design, she has a lifelong interest in how we develop and grow as individuals and in community.